Selective Mutism in Children
Second Edition

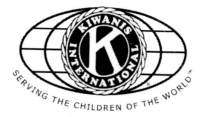

Selective Mutism in Children

Second Edition

by

Tony Cline BA, DipPsych
University of Luton

and

Sylvia Baldwin BA(Hons), MSc
Educational Psychologist, Oxford

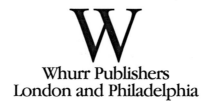

W

Whurr Publishers
London and Philadelphia

© 2004 Whurr Publishers Ltd
First published 2004
by Whurr Publishers Ltd
19b Compton Terrace
London N1 2UN
England

British Library Cataloguing in Publication Data

A catalogue record for this book is available from the British Library.

ISBN 1 86156 362 0

Typeset by Adrian McLaughlin, a@microguides.net

Contents

Preface

In the decade since the first edition of this book was published there have been important developments in the study and treatment of selective mutism. Understanding of the subject has improved more dramatically than in any period since the phenomenon was first recognized over a century ago. Our review of the literature has led to the addition of over 100 publications to the bibliography. In this new edition we report recent developments in medication and combined therapies. New findings on the links between social anxiety, biological and genetic factors and selective mutism are described. At the same time we remain committed to understanding this pattern of behaviour in its full social context in family and community and to employing behavioural approaches to intervention alongside other methods.

Readers who seek a non-technical introduction to understanding and helping selectively mute children may choose to concentrate on Chapters 1, 2, 3, 4, 7 and 8. Chapter 1 introduces the subject as a whole, Chapter 2 analyses the children and their context in more detail, Chapter 3 discusses how selective mutism develops, Chapter 4 focuses on the school setting, and Chapters 7 and 8 outline methods of treatment.

These core sections of the book are supplemented by an account of non–behavioural approaches for treating selectively mute children (Chapter 5), a history of behavioural approaches (Chapter 6) and a discussion of the methodology of research (Chapter 9). These three chapters (and in particular Chapter 9) are necessarily more technical than the rest of the book.

We are grateful to many colleagues for comments on the ideas put forward here and to Alice Sluckin for the model she has provided of work with parents and children. We wish specifically to acknowledge the assistance with this book of Jo Neale, whose meticulous work on updating our literature review on the subject laid the basis for the preparation of this edition. We have also greatly appreciated the patient support of Emily Spence who facilitated our communications over the work in progress.

Preface to first edition

The phenomenon of children who talk readily in some situations but not in others was recognised in the nineteenth century by the German physician, Kussmaul. The term elective mutism was coined by Tramer (1934) who offered the first full description. The phenomenon is rare, but it has generated a great deal of interest. Two years ago the guest editor of the journal *Educational and Child Psychology* commissioned us to prepare a short paper for educational psychologists on selective mutism (Baldwin and Cline, 1991). In working on that paper we found that the extensive and stimulating literature of papers in scientific and professional journals was not easily accessible and did not offer an overview. There was no up-to-date, book-length account of the subject in print. Thomas R. Kratochwill's 1981 text remains a rich source of information and ideas, but there have been important developments in the last decade which needed to be brought together in a single place. In addition, we wished to present a new model for understanding selective mutism in its full social context and a new strategy for selecting and implementing behavioural approaches to intervention. This book is the result.

Where individual children are described and no published reference is given, the account is taken from either Sylvia Baldwin's practice or correspondence received after an article on selective mutism in the *Times Educational Supplement*. In these cases names have been changed but the correspondents' own words have been used as far as possible. We are grateful to many colleagues for comments on the ideas put forward here, and we wish specifically to acknowledge the assistance of Patrick Leman in work on a draft research outline which laid the basis for the development of the Appendix, and of Anja Boeing who was responsible for the translation of key material from German.

Chapter 1
Introduction

Children who are selectively mute

He shows no sign of speaking at all. But he is very willing to complete tasks in his books; he is very neat and precise in his work. He can match 'like' words and pick out words I tell him to for reading. He loves listening to stories. However, he will not participate in any movement or games lessons and cries if I involve him. (He does enjoy watching though!) As far as I can tell from my experiences with him, he is extremely stubborn and very aware of what he is doing. He has told his mother (he speaks to all his family though not in school) that he will not speak until he is 7, and he obviously means to keep to it! He stopped speaking in nursery school when his parents were splitting up. Things have improved since he first started school. He will now give me eye contact when I am speaking to him and will carry out any tasks I ask him to. (Previously he would stand on one spot and refuse to do anything.) He will also go to the toilet with another child in the class. (Previously he would just wet his pants.) I am contriving to try open-ended questions with him, but he is very quick to realize when he has to give an answer and when he can nod to answer.

Reception class teacher on John (aged 5)

For the first time in 14 years of primary teaching I find myself with a child in my class who chooses not to speak to me. Lizzie is the youngest child of a family of three. Her older brother and sister have both been in my class and were both outgoing, talkative children. The family has had its problems. Father left the family although he has maintained contact and their mother has recently remarried. This does not have any bearing on Lizzie's behaviour since she has shown a similar pattern from an early age. She has not spoken to certain members of her family, particularly men, at all . . . (In the nursery) she was always prepared to join in with songs, poems, rhymes, etc, but she would not speak to the nursery teacher or nursery nurses. By the end of her time there (part-time education for approximately one and a half years) she would whisper one-word responses to direct questions. She usually had her finger in her mouth and did not use eye-to-eye contact . . . Now (in the reception class) she has progressed considerably . . . She is very

1

friendly with one or two other children, holds hands, giggles and laughs. She never asks when she needs something but will stand by my side until I guess what she wants . . . will now whisper one-word answers to my direct questions. My skill at lip reading is quickly improving! On one occasion she spoke loud enough for me to hear her across the width of a table. She will not speak to me if other children can hear her.

Reception class teacher about Lizzie (almost 5)

By the age of 6 she had established the reputation of not talking to any adult or any child in the school. She would communicate with her limited group of friends outside on the playground. She did 'accidentally' speak once or twice during the term and having realized immediately clammed up and avoided any kind of body contact. As she grew older the problem worsened in that the children always spoke for her, reinforcing the situation, and she would never establish eye contact. Her parents were not cooperative, as we saw it, not recognizing any problem.

Primary class teacher about Faith (aged 7)

. . . I refused to give in. As time went on, I became more and more resilient. I hated the teachers pestering me and saw them rather as the enemy. I had been at school for about three years and was beginning to think how nice it would be if I could communicate with the other children. I fancied having a special 'writing machine' rather like a typewriter. My parents meanwhile couldn't fathom me out, but since I was a perfectly normal child outside school, hoped it was just a phase. But my time was up. My mother suggested moving to a smaller (private) school. She told me solemnly that I would have to speak. Secretly I was dying to. I remember the first morning on the school bus. The prefect called out the register of the new girls and I remember the relief I felt – my stomach was churning – at answering 'yes'. You'll be pleased to know that from that time I was a typical giggly 8-year-old and am still talking nineteen to the dozen. I'm told I'm making up for those lost years.

Young adult recalling her own experience when
selectively mute between the ages of 4 and 8.

He stopped speaking to adults when his brother (2 years old) was born. Before this he had always been a shy child . . . Mrs S. told me some time later that when she was young she had experienced the same problems as Peter. Her family had moved house and she had to attend a new school in a new area. She did not speak at school for quite some time. She was then also worried that Peter's younger brother might develop the same problem. Both children and Mrs S. are extremely shy people.

Headteacher of a small rural primary school about Peter (aged 4)

It was almost as though we were talking about two different children, one at home and one at school, because Mrs P. said that at home Anita could be bossy with her younger sister, then aged 2, and rude and defiant towards her parents, whereas at school she seemed inhibited and conforming. Her mother did say, though, that she could be shy with people she did not know.

Home–school liaison teacher about Anita (aged 5)

The miracle has finally happened. James is now talking in the classroom. The breakthrough happened this morning but he has been nearing it for some time. He had written his story in his book, and the teacher asked him to read it. He started in a very hoarse voice, sort of spitting it out and then coughed. But he did it again, though in a very quiet voice. He got a special sticker and over the rest of the day started to speak in his ordinary voice. The teacher did remember not to make a great fuss about it, and I'm sure this helped.

And 6 months later:

He is a different boy now at home. He asks questions in class and isn't afraid to approach the Head if he wants to tell her something. At the end of the day I sometimes have to drag him out of the cloakroom because I want to get home.

The mother of James (aged 5) who had been mute since nursery school

I came to feel very disappointed and at a loss when she would not speak, merely pull ridiculous faces as a reply to my questions and attempts to converse. I found it very frustrating not to get any response at all, however hard I tried and whatever tactics I employed . . . Jane talked to her neighbour, who then translated her needs or what she had said. In the playground she played with a group of girls but was the one who always went last or broke the rules . . . at the end of a lesson, particularly lunchtime, Jane would often run through the classroom shouting and looking at me as if to tell me that she did have a voice but chose not to honour me with it.

Student on teaching practice about Jane (aged 10)

In extremes some children withdraw speech from members of their family too. Wallace (1986) gave a vivid description of mealtimes with silent twins, June and Jennifer:

They turned the Gibbons' chatty family table into a Trappist refectory. Direct questions asked at mealtimes received no acknowledgement except an occasional nod. The twins took no part in family discussions but bowed their heads, eyes fixed on their plates, their faces without expression, tight and drawn in denial of the world around them. To Aubrey, Greta and David they would not utter even a syllable, but they did talk and play with Rosie, the baby of the family.

As those accounts illustrate, there is considerable variation in the behaviour associated with selective mutism, but there are also certain key elements that are shared. The children persist in silence with all adults (and sometimes with other children) in certain settings outside the home; they develop non-verbal strategies for communicating their needs and getting their way; they appear shy and sensitive, but also watchful, stubborn and devious; they can behave in an assertive, even a bold fashion while still not speaking; they generate strong feelings of frustration and anger in the adults to whom they refuse to speak. This is the pattern of behaviour that is the subject of this book. It is rather rare, which makes it even more of a challenge for competent teachers, speech therapists and nursery staff. They have to develop strategies for tackling an extremely difficult management problem without the benefit of prior experience. They often feel isolated as well as frustrated. Even the professionals who might be expected to offer support in such situations will have very limited experience on which to draw. A survey of educational psychologists in East Sussex indicated that on average they had encountered a selectively mute child once every five years (Buck, 1988). This estimate has been confirmed in anecdotal evidence from educational psychologists working in other areas (Imich, 1998). In a series of 2250 referrals to the schools psychological service and child guidance services in Wiltshire only four children were described as selectively mute (Clayton, 1981). Paediatricians too receive referrals of this group very rarely (see commentary by Yapko in Stein et al., 2001), and family doctors rarely report them, except in areas of high immigration (Shvartzman et al., 1990). (See later in the chapter – 'Incidence of selective mutism' – for a more detailed discussion of incidence.)

Thus the rarity of this pattern of behaviour adds to the difficulties it presents to adults trying to help. One of our aims in this book is to suggest strategies for assessment and treatment that 'normalize' the pattern by allowing early intervention without the child or the family being labelled as deviant and by making clear what further steps are possible if the initial attempts to help are unsuccessful. In adopting this approach we do not wish to minimize the challenge that selective mutism presents. It is easy to do that: someone meeting any of the children described above for the first time might have thought of them as just a little shy and might initially have imagined that they would 'soon get over it', that they 'could speak if they wanted to', that it was 'only a phase'. All too often in the case histories outlined by teachers someone is reported to have given somewhat misleading advice along these lines. Time alone, they said, would effect a cure. It was often implied that this would not require any modification of the behaviour of others towards the child. In fact, however, once a pattern of mutism is established it can be very resistant to change. It is important to address the problem directly and to ensure that the response of those around the child is not reinforcing the pattern. The starting point must be to define what the problem is.

The definition of selective mutism

Selective mutism occurs when children are able to speak and do speak in some situations (e.g. with some members of their family) but persist in remaining silent when interacting with some other people in some other settings. There are variations, but this statement sets out the core features of what is properly known as selective mutism. A useful reference point for discussion is the short statement on diagnostic criteria in the latest version of the American Psychiatric Association's diagnostic guide, *Diagnostic and Statistical Manual of Mental Disorders*, 4th edition (DSM-IV) (APA, 1994). In an earlier edition of this guide the first criterion was 'persistent refusal to talk in one or more major social situations (including at school)'. The words 'persistent refusal' were revised to 'consistent failure' in the fourth edition in order to avoid implying that it is assumed that children are being oppositional or obstinate when they remain silent. The possibility is left open that their failure to speak may result from fear or anxiety (Rapoport and Ismond, 1996).

Table 1.1 Diagnostic criteria for selective mutism according to DSM-IV (APA, 1994)

Consistent failure to speak in specific social situations (in which there is an expectation for speaking, e.g. at school) despite speaking in other situations

The disturbance interferes with educational or occupational achievement or with social communication

The duration of the disturbance is at least 1 month (not limited to the first month of school)

The failure to speak is not due to a lack of knowledge of, or comfort with, the spoken language required in the social situation

The disturbance is not better accounted for by a communication disorder (e.g. stuttering) and does not occur exclusively during the course of a pervasive developmental disorder, schizophrenia or other psychotic disorder

The child's failure to speak in some situations is 'consistent'. For the term *selective mutism* to be applied the behaviour must interfere with educational or occupational achievement or with social communication and must last for at least one month (more than one month when beginning school). Many children go through phases of reticence when getting used to a novel situation. Their behaviour is not usefully described as selective mutism, because its course of development is quite different and it may need to be managed in a different way. Even so some writers have used the term elective mutism for a transitory reaction (e.g. Chapel, 1970). There is room for debate as to how long selective silence has to last before it is helpful to think of it as conforming to the pattern of selective mutism. Initially we suspected that the DSM-IV prescription of 'at least 1 month' was too short. Brown and Lloyd (1975) studied a cohort of children starting school in Birmingham in one year. The majority of children who were silent when they started at school had begun to speak within 32–40 weeks. Out of a total of 6072 children, 42 were not speaking after 8 weeks, 4 after 32 weeks and 1 after 64 weeks. Kolvin and Fundudis (1981) used a criterion of persistence over two years at this age level, and one year if a child's mutism started when they were older (cf. Silverman and Powers, 1970). The two-year criterion seems highly restrictive. It implies that there is a good prospect of change in the second year, an optimism which does not seem to have any substantial basis in the literature. Yet, if this criterion is used, children are likely to be left for an extended period before any systematic effort is made to help them overcome their difficulties.

Bradley and Sloman (1975) employed the criterion of mute behaviour for a whole school year for their survey in Canada. Taking account of the pattern seen in Brown and Lloyd's statistics in Table 1.2 and of clinical experience as reflected in the literature, in the first edition of this book we suggested that within the age range 5–7 years persistence over a period of six months or two school terms should be seen as sufficient to justify thinking of a child as selectively mute. If a carefully considered programme of assessment and treatment is employed, we thought, there would be no risk of intervening more heavily than is required with children whose mutism has lasted that long (see Chapter 7). The same criterion had been used by Wright et al. (1985) and Wilkins (1985). If a child were older than 7, we suggested, there might well be justification for a shorter criterion period than six months, e.g. one month as proposed in DSM-IV (APA, 1994).

Table 1.2 Number of children not speaking at school during their first year

No. of weeks after start of school year	8	16	24	32	40	56	64	72
No. of children not speaking	42	29	15	5	4	2	1	1

From Brown and Lloyd (1975).

There is one serious disadvantage in adopting a period of six months' non-speaking as the criterion for describing a child as selectively mute. This may avoid the risk of a false positive error – diagnosing selective mutism when the child is just taking a long time to settle into a new situation, and thus pathologizing a transient difficulty unnecessarily. But, if the child really is developing long-term problems of communication, it is unhelpful to postpone intervention at this stage. As will be clear in Chapter 4, we advocate a 'light touch' preventive strategy in nurseries and schools. This should enable teachers and other staff to support children in overcoming initial difficulties of communication without making them into a 'patient' or treating their pattern of behaviour as 'pathological'. It is always important to take account of a child's history of speaking (and not speaking) in earlier settings or at home. The date of referral for help may be much later than the date of onset, which, as noted below, may be insidious. With that proviso we accept the DSM-IV definition that is coming into general use – that a child should be described as selectively mute if the duration of non-speaking in a setting outside the home is at least one month (except when that is their first month at school).

Selective mutism and shyness

Children who refuse to speak in some situations are often seen as shy. In a survey of 30 children with selective mutism Black and Uhde (1995) found that 23% of their parents described them as 'somewhat shy', 20% as 'moderately shy' and 57% as 'extremely shy' (p. 850). In a larger survey of 100 children Steinhausen and Juzi (1996) found that 85% had been rated as 'shy' by those who knew them. Sometimes being 'just a little shy' is seen as the only problem that a child with selective mutism has. This is misleading: shyness may often be one of the characteristics of a child with selective mutism, but it is never the whole story. It is important to differentiate the ordinary shyness that is within the normal range of variation in personal temperament from the exceptional pattern of development represented by selective mutism. There are a number of reasons for emphasizing this distinction – notably, marked differences in aetiology, in the course of development once a particular pattern of responding is established, and in the most beneficial approaches to support or intervention.

There has been a substantial increase in research in shyness in recent years. Increasingly shyness is seen as a complex phenomenon that presents differently in young children from its form in older children and adults. Young children will show *fearful* shyness characterized by timidity and wariness, while those who are older will show *self-conscious* shyness characterized by embarrassment and concern about how others judge them (Crozier, 2002). Shyness is relatively common. In one large-scale survey nearly all respondents reported that they felt shy sometimes and 40% described themselves as shy. Selective mutism, on the other hand, is less common and is defined in terms of observable behaviour rather than self-report. There may be a biological and genetic basis to both phenomena, but they show quite different patterns of development. Unlike shyness, selective mutism as a pattern of behaviour is socially disabling to such a degree that it requires direct intervention. Underlying traits of behavioural inhibition and anxiety play a part in the development of both phenomena. In recent years there have been important advances in thinking about the role that anxiety plays in underpinning the development of selective mutism and maintaining the pattern of behaviour once it has developed (Leonard and Dow, 1995; Anstendig, 1999). These advances will be discussed in detail in Chapters 2 and 3.

Differentiating selective mutism from other kinds of mutism

Selective mutism, which is assumed to have its origins in the child's social and emotional development, has to be differentiated from mute behaviour that has a quite different basis. Some children who are mute do not talk in any setting. Their mutism is associated with an organic condition such as aphasia or deafness. Mutism sometimes occurs as one of the features associated with autism or childhood schizophrenia (Gillberg, 1996) or pervasive refusal syndrome (Taylor et al., 2000). There is no difficulty in these cases in distinguishing the children's persistent mutism from the pattern of communication in selective mutism.

In general, in the same way, it is not difficult to discriminate between Asperger's syndrome and autism on the one hand and selective mutism on the other. As Graham et al. (1999) pointed out, 'the possibility of autism is excluded by the child showing affectionate social relationships at home and the use of gesture to express needs and to share interests at school' (p. 78). However, there are some overlapping symptoms: both groups of children show social anxiety and, often, fear of the unfamiliar. They may therefore cling to established habits. Thus, in rare cases, a child may show both patterns of difficulty (e.g. Robbie in Johnson and Wintgens, 2001, p. 221). More commonly, because of the current tendency to over-diagnose Asperger's syndrome (Selfe 2002), selective mutism may be confusingly diagnosed as Asperger's syndrome when there is no strong evidence of the latter. The risk in that situation is that an intervention that could have succeeded in helping the child towards a more normal everyday pattern of communication will not be attempted.

It has been argued that the use of symbols by selectively mute children is so atypical that their problems should be considered as similar to those of children with 'more severe psychotic-spectrum disorders' (Atlas, 1993, p. 1079), but the evidence presented in support of this view was not convincing and all other writers on the subject have taken a different view. There has also been one report of a link between selective mutism and dissociative identity disorder (Jacobsen, 1995), but, again, there has been no corroboration of such a link by any other investigators.

There have been very rare reports of selective mutism persisting into adolescence and then becoming one aspect of an incipient schizophrenic or schizoid episode (Youngerman, 1979; Eldar et al., 1985). In such cases it has sometimes appeared that a key factor in the deterioration was mismanagement of the initial pattern of deviant behaviour. Hayden (1983) and Wallace (1986) provide vivid anecdotal illustrations of this process. But other children whose selective mutism persists into adolescence have not experienced extreme problems or complicating factors (e.g. the 14-year-old boy described by Lysne, 1995), and we have noted that no recent reports have confirmed the alarming pictures drawn by writers such as Youngerman.

A different developmental sequence involves a young person becoming selectively mute in early adolescence and then developing a range of more extreme symptoms of severe emotional disturbance (Kaplan and Escoll, 1973). In all these cases there is a clear period in the child's development when the main presenting symptom is selective mutism. The development of other extreme symptoms comes later. A similar pattern was reported by Albert-Stewart (1986) and Tibbles and Russell (1992). This sequence can be distinguished without difficulty from the situation in which mutism is one of a number of causes for concern presenting simultaneously in a child with autism or schizophrenia.

Does the child speak in any setting?

If children are observed to be mute in some settings, the next point to be established is that they can speak and be understood in other settings. Their speech may be immature or laboured or difficult to follow, but those to whom they choose to speak can follow what they are saying. Some writers in the past have used the term inappropriately for children who did not speak in any situation (e.g. Adams and Glasner, 1954; Blake and Moss, 1967). Some selectively mute children have abnormalities of speech (or believe they do). The critical point is that they can communicate with some people but do not use the verbal abilities they have with everyone they might be expected to speak to. That is why their mutism is described as elective or selective.

Does the child have learning difficulties?

Some children fail to speak because of severe or profound learning difficulties that affect all aspects of their development. They do not use speech with anyone. Some children with less severe learning difficulties achieve effective verbal communication over familiar content areas with those with whom they have regular contact and who understand them best. They may need these people to be present to facilitate speech with those who are less familiar with them and in new situations. Their failure to speak in some situations does not constitute selective mutism in the sense used here. However, distinguishing them may present more of a challenge than in cases of deafness and aphasia. Many authors have set firm IQ limits to clarify the position. For example, Wilkins (1985) in his review of a series of hospital medical notes admitted into the elective mute sample only children who, as well as meeting the other criteria, had an IQ of 70 or more on the Wechsler Intelligence Scale for Children (compare Silverman and Powers, 1970; Hayden, 1980.) There are strong arguments against exclusion solely on the basis of IQ (see fuller discussion later in this chapter – 'Intelligence'). The rationale underlying this criterion for those authors who include it is that the child's mutism should not arise solely because of retarded mental development. This is the critical issue: it is reasonable to think of children whose intelligence is limited, but who only communicate readily to some people or in some settings, as selectively mute because they can be helped by the methods employed for selective mutism (compare APA, 1994, p. 115).

There are also rare examples of children with sensory disabilities becoming selectively mute. For example, Kass et al. (1967) described a blind girl aged 6 who had remained silent throughout nursery school and kindergarten. There was no suggestion that her sensory disability caused her selective mutism, though obviously it affected both how it was manifested and how it could be treated (compare Brown and Doll, 1988).

Is the child's mutism a temporary reaction to trauma or tragic events?

Selective mutism is assumed to have its roots in emotional difficulties. Most of us are familiar with the idea that a failure of speech can arise from acute stress, as in stage fright or in the state of shock that follows a sudden disaster such as a fire or a tornado (Elson et al., 1965). Such lapses are temporary and normally short-lived. Szabo (1996) described the reactions of a 5-year-old black South African girl whose family had not fully explained to her what had happened to her mother who had, in fact, been murdered some weeks earlier. She ceased to speak to her family. The psychiatric team's brief and successful intervention was to help the family to communicate the truth to her and encourage them to take her on a visit to the grave site.

Adults find it easy to empathize with a child who is shy for a limited period in an unfamiliar situation. It is not difficult to appreciate the threat in the situation and the stress it causes the child. But it is assumed that the novelty will soon wear off and that the child will be able to interact more and more normally as that happens. So-called 'traumatic mutism' persists only very rarely (Kolvin and Fundudis, 1981; Black and Uhde, 1995), and surveys of selectively mute children show no association between traumatic experience and the development of their communication problems (Steinhausen and Juzi, 1996). However, parents of a selectively mute child will often single out an important early event in his or her life as particularly traumatic and trace the mutism back to it. Yanof (1996) argued that trauma may have been underreported because 'the patient usually cannot report, and what may be traumatic to a young child may not be recognized easily by the adults in his world' (p. 81). Andersson and Thomsen (1998) noted that over a third of the hospital case records of selective mutism that they reviewed had a reference to a traumatic event in the child's early life, but they argued that, as the information had not been assessed in a consistent way at the time of interview, its aetiological significance could not be evaluated. 'It is possible that the parents were specifically asked about traumatic events, and this may explain the large number' (p. 237). Although some writers have claimed that psychological trauma can be an important factor (e.g. Kolakowski, Liwska and Wolanczyk, 1996) and there are some persuasive individual case studies (e.g. Valner and Nemiroff, 1995), this view has very little support in the literature.

It appears to be easier to accept the stance of the mute child whose emotional resistance to speaking is 'justified' by a traumatic experience and lasts for only a short time. When there is no apparent 'justification' and the refusal to speak is selective and persistent, there is often disagreement as to whether the child is being stubborn and self-willed or is somehow incapacitated by emotional forces beyond her* control. The reactions of adults to a selectively mute child are to some extent influenced by their moral judgment on such questions. This issue is of some

---

* For convenience, we use the female form of the pronoun to refer to selectively mute children at various points in the text.

importance in planning intervention. It will be discussed further in Chapter 2. (There are other forms of mutism with psychogenic or emotional roots, though they are even more uncommon in childhood than selective mutism and will not be discussed here, e.g. 'hysterical aphonia' and hysterical conversion reactions mentioned by Akhtar and Buckman, 1977.)

Differentiating within selective mutism

Some of the debate on definitions in this field has focused not on differentiating selective mutism from other conditions but on differentiating various conditions *within* selective mutism. For example, an important issue for some writers has been whether the child talks at all in the situation in which she is normally mute. Williamson et al. (1977b), Morin, Ladouceur and Cloutier (1982) and Hill and Scull (1985) have been at pains to distinguish 'reluctant speech' from selective mutism. In the former condition the child may talk to peers in the classroom but not to the teacher, or may talk to the teacher briefly in some circumstances but not otherwise (e.g. reading aloud from a book). Where this limited speech occurs in such circumstances, a simpler form of behavioural intervention is possible. So it is important to identify the fact, and these authors choose to give this pattern of behaviour a different name. Others (e.g. Straughan, Potter and Hamilton, 1965; Brown and Doll, 1988) have simply used the term *elective mutism*. But there is a temptation to develop an increasing number of different terms to distinguish slightly different conditions under the general heading of selective mutism.

Another illustration of this tendency is a paper by Paniagua and Saeed (1988). They highlighted the situation in which a child who is already selectively mute outside the family progressively reduces verbal interactions with family members too. Such cases are very rare, but they were able to identify four in the literature. One of us (SB) has noted two children who reacted to their parents' increasing concern about their mutism outside by temporarily becoming resistant to speaking at home too. In each case this was a short-lived pattern and did not require specific clinical attention. The term *progressive mutism* is misleading, since the rare cases of mutism at home do not normally follow a period of selective mutism outside (Wilkins, 1985). Paniagua and Saeed argue that it is important to make a differential diagnosis between selective and progressive mutism in order to plan behavioural intervention appropriately. It is certainly true that the planning of behavioural intervention requires a detailed analysis of which people the child speaks to in which settings. But we do not consider it helpful to multiply 'diagnostic' terms for this purpose. A more direct and straightforward assessment strategy is preferable (see Chapter 7). In general, we favour a broad, overarching, atheoretical, descriptive term for the phenomena of selective mutism. This seems to lay the best possible foundation for full understanding and effective management and treatment. (Compare the discussion of 'behavioral diagnosis of mutism' in Kratochwill, 1981, Chapter 1.)

At the same time it is important to acknowledge the heterogeneity of the group of children who present with selective mutism. Authors vary in how they react to this. For example, Wright (1968) hesitated to use the term because of the variety within his clinical sample of 24 children, and Bhide and Srinath (1985) argued that inadequacies in some reported research meant that the case for 'a distinct clinical syndrome' had not been made. Atoynatan (1986) excluded from her series of cases of selectively mute children one child with an articulation defect and another who spoke to no one other than his mother and a sister. Hayden (1980), on the other hand, courted criticism because she included an exceptionally wide range in a large sample of 68 children whom she firmly called elective mutes (Kolvin and Fundudis, 1981). But even those who have adopted a tight definition for what constitutes elective mutism have found considerable heterogeneity within the sample (e.g. Koch and Goodlund, 1973). In Chapter 2 we will discuss suggestions that have been made for classifying subtypes of the condition in more detail.

Elective mutism or selective mutism? The choice of terms

Selective mutism is one of a number of ways in which children show 'restricted speech' during their development (Schill, Kratochwill and Gardner (1996b), p. 103). A wide variety of terms has been used for the phenomena associated specifically with selective mutism. Kratochwill (1981) listed the following:

elective mutism	functional mutism
hearing mute	negativism
selective mutism	speech avoidance
speech inhibition	speech phobia
speech shyness	suppressed speech
thymogenic mutism	temporary mutism
voluntary mutism	

It might have been hoped that consensual support for a single term would develop in the years following Kratochwill's major review. In the event new terms have continued to appear to enliven the picture:

- situation-specific mutism (Conrad, Delk and Williams, 1974)
- psychogenic mutism (Mack and Maslin, 1981)
- psychological mutism (Paniagua and Saeed, 1987)
- voluntary silence (Louden, 1987)
- silence users (Hadley, 1994)
- restricted speech (Schill, Kratochwill and Gardner, 1996b).

Few of the terms have a distinct meaning or separate rationale (though the last in that list highlights the fact that silence itself may carry a message – see Chapter 2). The term that was used most often over the years was *elective mutism*. But a consensus slowly developed that *selective mutism* was preferable (APA, 1994). That term seems to capture the key features of the phenomenon most clearly: it is selective and it involves a lack of speech where speech is normally found. A particular advantage of this term is that it does not introduce any untested assumptions into the labelling of the behaviour. For example, it does not imply that children elect or choose to remain silent, and it does not automatically associate their pattern of behaviour with a phobic reaction. Although *elective mutism* continued to be very widely used for many years, a number of other writers preferred the alternative term (e.g. Kass et al., 1967; Reid et al., 1967; Rasbury, 1974; Kratochwill, 1981). The use of *selective mutism* in the DSM-IV Manual (APA, 1994) is likely to prove decisive in the long term. (We ourselves, though, see some advantages in the use of the term *restricted speech*, because it avoids the stigmatizing connotations of 'mutism'.) Whatever term is chosen, it is essential to use the category label in a precise way. But in planning work with an individual child labelling remains less important than describing the child's behaviour precisely: to whom does she talk, in which situations and settings, how often, how loudly, with what confidence and fluency, and for how long?

Incidence of selective mutism

Overall incidence

The rarity of this phenomenon has determined to a large extent how its incidence has been studied. The most common form of report in the literature has been an analysis of the proportion of children seen in a single clinic or centre who are diagnosed as selectively mute. These reports emphasize the low frequency of the phenomenon. A summary is presented in Table 1.3.

In large hospital departments in urban areas the modal incidence of selective mutism referrals appears to be in the region of 0.5% of all referrals of children and adolescents, but there is considerable variation. This may be accounted for in three ways:

- Different teams employed different criteria for selective mutism. The highest frequencies in that list are associated with reports in which the criterion used is not stated or is very broad (e.g. Wright, 1968).
- Some workers and centres become known for their expertise in helping clients with particular kinds of problem. The number of referrals of that kind of problem may then increase (Wright, 1968; Johnson and Wintgens, 2001, p. 28).
- There is reason to believe that the phenomenon may be more common in families who are socially isolated either in rural communities or as

Table 1.3 Incidence of selective mutism in referrals in child psychology and psychiatry

Source	Number of cases	% referrals
Andersson and Thomsen (1998)	37 cases out of approx. 7000 records of referrals to a psychiatric hospital for Children and Adolescents in Aarhus, Denmark	approx. 0.5
Browne, Wilson and Laybourne (1963)	10 cases in a 12-year period in the child psychiatry facility of University of Kansas Medical Center	
Clayton (1981)	4 of 2250 school psychological service and child guidance referrals in Wiltshire, England	0.18
Kolvin and Fundudis (1981)	24 children over a period of 5–6 years in all child psychiatry and child guidance clinics in the area of Newcastle, England	
Krohn, Weckstein and Wright (1992)[a]	20 cases out of 3939 seen at the Hawthorn Centre, Northville, Michigan over the period 1978–1992	0.5
Lesser-Katz (1986)	8 Head Start children in one year and 7 the next year from a school of 88 in Chicago	
Looff (1971)	10 of 287 children reviewed in the field clinics of the Manchester Project in Eastern Kentucky over the period 1964–70; also 2 of 113 Eastern Kentucky children reviewed at a university medical center over the period 1964–68	2.8 1.6
Morris (1953)	6 of 600 cases seen over a 3-year period in child guidance clinics in Norfolk, Virginia	1
Parker, Olsen and Throckmorton (1960)	27 of 3600 children referred to school social workers in Tacoma, Washington, over a 12-year period	0.75
Pustrom and Speers (1964)	3 children over a 9–10-year period seen at the Child Psychiatry Unit of the North Carolina Memorial Hospital	
Reed (1963)	4 of 2000 city and urban children referred to a large English child guidance clinic	0.2
Salfield (1950)	2 out of 'more than an estimated 500 child guidance cases' reported from Dumfries, Scotland	maximum 0.4

continued

Table 1.3 continued

Source	Number of cases	% referrals
Silverman and Powers (1970)	5 children seen over a period of 8 years at the Virginia Treatment Center for Children in Richmond, Virginia	
Steinhausen and Juzi (1996)	59 children out of 12,438 seen between 1979 and 1992 in the Child and Adolescent Psychiatric Service of Zurich, Switzerland	
Wilkins (1985)	22 patients out of 4,093 seen at a University Department of Child and Adolescent Psychiatry in Berlin between 1978 and 1985	
Wright (1968)	24 cases over a 12-year period at the Children's Dept of the Maudsley Hospital, London (excluding cases where either parent was not a fluent English speaker)	0.47
	24 children referred over a 7-year period to a large psychiatric clinic in Northville, Michigan for refusal to talk at school	0.54
Wright et al. (1985)	4 of 61 preschool children seen at a diagnostic nursery admitting relatively severe psychiatric referrals in a metropolitan area in South Carolina	6.5

[a] Wright, 1968, covers the same clinic during an earlier period.

immigrants in multiethnic areas of large cities. Relatively high frequencies may be identified with clinics or counsellors positioned to receive a relatively high proportion of such families (e.g. Morris, 1953; Lesser-Katz, 1986; compare Looff, 1971, pp. 84–85; Calhoun and Koenig, 1973).

It is not possible to extrapolate from figures for prevalence in clinic populations to estimate the incidence in the whole child population. For this a different kind of survey is necessary. There have been a small number of surveys of school populations designed to determine incidence. Until recently all had been in urban areas. Their results are shown in Table 1.4, with comments on three factors that may have influenced their findings on prevalence rates – the age range of the population studied, the criteria employed for selective mutism, and the proportion of immigrant, ethnic minority or bilingual children in the population. (It will be noted that this last figure is not always stated and has had to be inferred in some cases.)

It will be seen that the ratio figures quoted in published studies are inconsistent. When we wrote the first edition of this book 10 years ago,

Table 1.4 Population surveys of the incidence of selective mutism

Researchers	Population characteristics	Criteria	Ratio of selectively mute children
Bradley and Sloman (1975)	School population of Toronto, Canada (6,865 aged 5–12 years, 64–76% immigrant or non-English speaking)	Not speaking persisted for 12 months	3 : 1000[a]
Brown and Lloyd (1975)	School population of Birmingham, UK (6072 children aged 5 followed through their first 72 weeks at school. School population appears to have had 33% ethnic minorities)	Not speaking persisted for 6 or 12 months	0.8 : 1000 if criterion was 6 months 0.33–0.66 : 1000 if criterion was 12 months
Fundudis, Kolvin and Garside (1979)	Total birth cohort of 3,300 children studied longitudinally in Newcastle, UK. Report based on follow-up at the age of 7. Proportion of immigrant and ethnic minority pupils not stated but appears to have been low	Mutism persisting to the seventh year	0.6 : 1000[b]
Kopp and Gillberg (1997)	School population of two school districts of Goteborg, Sweden aged 7–15 years (2793 pupils)	DSM-IV	1.8 : 1000
Kumpulainen et al. (1998)	School population in second grade of Kuopio County, Finland (2,434 pupils). Area had no pupils from ethnic or linguistic minorities	DSM-III-R	16 : 1000
Bergman, Piacentini and McCracken (2002)	125 out of 133 kindergarten, first and second grade teachers from the 10 elementary schools constituting a public school district in Los Angeles. They considered 2,256 pupils	DSM-IV	7.1 : 1000

[a] 21 selectively mute children identified.
[b] The authors state: 'We . . . consider 0.8 per 1000 as a minimum prevalence rate particularly as there remains the theoretical possibility that electively mute children could have slipped through our screen at the 3-year-old stage.'

we considered that the best estimate of incidence was the one on which Brown and Lloyd (1975) and Fundudis, Kolvin and Garside (1979) agreed – 0.8 per 1000 employing a '6 months' persistence' criterion in defining selective mutism. We suggested that the ratio would be higher in urban areas where there is a high proportion of immigrant or ethnic minority families and in rural areas where there is a high proportion of families living in isolated situations. However, we acknowledged that under-reporting might upset these calculations. After reviewing the literature Hesselman (1983) commented: 'Personally I support those who claim that there are probably many hidden cases' (p. 299). Similarly Kopp and Gillberg (1997) defended their higher estimate of incidence by pointing out that parents often do not see a selectively mute pattern of behaviour as problematic and so seek help 'only after considerable "pressure" from teachers and others' (p. 260).

The exceptionally high incidence found by Kumpulainen et al. (1998) requires some explanation. They sought to confirm the reliability of the teacher reports by asking school health nurses to check them. This seems to have been a less rigorous procedure than employed by Kopp and Gillberg who undertook the checking directly themselves and followed it up over a period of a year. In addition, the definition of selective mutism used in the Finnish study was the DSM-III-R criteria (APA, 1987) which were looser than the DSM-IV criteria used in the Swedish study. There was a further crucial factor: Kumpulainen et al. focused on children in second grade, but Kopp and Gillberg surveyed a much wider age range. The reporting of selective mutism is at its height after school entry, so that focusing on second grade was likely to yield a higher incidence rate. The discrepancy between this study and all others is so substantial that it is difficult to give it too much credence without further evidence.

Bergman, Piacentini and McCracken (2002) published the first report of a population study in the USA. They surveyed teachers of kindergarten, first and second grade classes in the 10 elementary schools in a single school district in Los Angeles. Children who did not speak English fluently were excluded from the study. They found a prevalence rate of 0.71% employing the DSM-IV criteria for selective mutism. On follow-up six months later three of the seven kindergarten pupils showed 'notable improvements in SM symptoms' (p. 943). This study suggests an incidence rate in the first three years of full-time schooling that is greater than we had accepted in the first edition of this book, though not as great as that reported by Kumpulainen et al. (1998).

Taking account of this survey and of the argument set out earlier, we have come to share their view that the incidence rate usually quoted is an underestimate. There is one further piece of evidence to support that claim. When individual professionals or centres are known to take a particular interest in selective mutism, they receive more referrals than would be possible with the proposed incidence figure (e.g. Wright, 1968;

Lesser-Katz, 1986). A further factor has been suggested that may be leading to an increase in the reported incidence. As many societies such as the
United States admit children to preschool and nursery programmes at
younger ages, 'increased numbers of children [i.e children with selective
mutism] will be uncovered' (Joseph, 1999, p. 309). For the present it
seems reasonable to adopt an estimate of 6–8 cases of selective mutism
per 1000 children through childhood with certain conditions but to
remain open to the possibility that that may well be an underestimate.
More population studies of the type undertaken in Toronto, Birmingham,
Newcastle, Goteborg, Kuopio and Los Angeles would help to resolve the
question.

Gender

For most types of language difficulty in childhood, incidence is higher
among boys than among girls. It is generally agreed that selective mutism
is unusual in that it is found at least as frequently, if not more frequently,
among girls. This has caused a good deal of comment and discussion.
Haenel and Werder, two Swiss child psychiatrists, are cited by Hesselman
(1983) as claiming that 'nothing supports the suggested opinions frequently published that girls dominate'. Subsequent reviews have provided
that support. Wright et al. (1985) and Lebrun (1990) analysed a large number of published studies. Their data are listed in Table 1.5 together with
evidence from studies up to 1993 that was not covered in their reviews. Of
302 children described in 98 reports published before 1993 57% were girls
and 43% boys. Subsequent surveys have confirmed this result. There
appears to be no doubt now that girls become selectively mute more often
than boys. Estimates of the preponderance of girls vary but tend to fall
within the range 55–65%. For example, Steinhausen and Juzi (1996) found
that girls comprised 62% of their sample of 100 selectively mute children,
and Krohn, Weckstein and Wright (1992) found that the proportion in
their sample of 20 children was 60%. That proportion was also found in
the population survey by Kopp and Gillberg (1997); Kumpulainen et al.
(1998) found 61% in the Finnish study, and Kristensen (2000) 59% in the
Norwegian survey. Higher proportions of girls have been reported by a
smaller number of researchers, including Wilkins (1985), Black and Uhde
(1995) and Ford et al. (1998), and higher proportions of boys by very few,
including Andersson and Thomsen (1998).

Why should selective mutism be an exception to the general finding
that language-related difficulties are more common in boys? Lebrun
(1990) commented simply that the reason was not known. Wilkins (1985)
linked this finding to age of onset: 'emotional disorders are commoner in
preschool girls than in boys'. In a commentary within the same tradition
Kolvin and Fundudis (1981) suggested that girls might be 'more vulnerable to excess of temperamental abnormalities, especially where there is a
familial predisposition to problems of social relationships.' It is certainly

Table 1.5 Gender of selectively mute children described in the literature up to 1993

Reference source	No. of studies reviewed	Boys	Girls
Wright et al. (1985)	47	35	44
Lebrun (1990)	9	38	56
Cline and Baldwin[a]	42	56	71
Total	98	129 (43%)	171 (57%)

[a] Unpublished data. List of references available from the first author.

a common observation that other family members besides the selectively mute child often have restricted social relationships or a quiet manner with others (see Chapter 2). The notion of some kind of familial predisposition has a theoretical basis in much recent work on childhood temperament (Prior, 1992). The notion that any familial predisposition might be sex-linked is open to empirical investigation. But no such study has been attempted in relation to selective mutism, and, even if genetic factors play some part in determining this phenomenon, it seems probable that cultural factors also play a significant role.

A number of writers have speculated about the process by which cultural factors might contribute to determining that selective mutism is found more often in girls than in boys. Within the psychodynamic tradition Meijer (1979) drew attention to the cultural taboo on girls expressing aggression openly when young. He suggested that for this reason they may be more prone to develop a hostile dependency on one parent, particularly the mother. There is some supporting evidence for this kind of process in single case reports in the psychodynamic literature (see Chapter 5), but no analysis has been carried out to test the hypothesis that girls may show such mechanisms more than boys. Of course, the behavioural tradition can also offer speculative ideas as to how the sex difference arises. For example, there is evidence in the clinical literature that some selectively mute girls adopt a pattern of behaviour that is congruent with the role model set by their mothers (e.g. Linda in Scott, 1977). This process can readily be explained within the framework of social learning theory.

Hayden (1980) reported an interesting observation about her large, rather loosely defined sample of selectively mute children: boys were referred on average 2.3 years earlier than girls. She suggested that this might be because passive, clinging, shy behaviour is tolerated in girls more than boys (p. 131). Hayden's sample was heterogeneous and included children who would not be termed selectively mute by the criteria we have employed in this book. So it would be of considerable interest to examine her hypothesis against clinical data reported by others. Her suggestion would be supported if evidence emerged that boys who present as selectively mute are referred for help at an earlier age than girls though the age of onset of their mutism is no different. That would support the contention that differential adult reactions to the same pattern of behaviour may play a significant role in the phenomenon. One problem is that, although all case studies report the age of referral, they do not all report the age of onset. In any case such reports are dependent on recollection by members of the family and may be differentially distorted for boys and girls. (For comments on other problems involved in defining age of onset see below.) Keeping these provisos in mind, we carried out a preliminary analysis of selected data in the table in Wright et al. (1985) which, as noted above, summarized information from 47 published case studies (Table 1.6). We concentrated on children who had presented as selectively mute by the age of 8. A number of cases were omitted from the analysis because of incomplete information (e.g. on age at first referral). We also excluded four unusual cases (all girls) where there had been an unexplained delay of 8–10 years between onset and referral. After these exclusions there were 23 boys and 21 girls.

As will be seen from the table, the girls became selectively mute when they were a few months younger on average than the boys and were

Table 1.6 Gender, age of onset and age of referral for selective mutism

	No. of cases	Reported age of onset (mean)	Age on first referral (years)	Difference (months)
Boys	23	4.6	6.9	27
Girls	21	4.1	7.3	38

referred for help when they were a few months older. The mean interval before referral for girls was 10 months longer than for boys (38 months as against 27 months). A more thorough analysis of a larger sample of cases is required, but these data offer preliminary support for Hayden's hypothesis. However, Ford et al. (1998) found no difference between girls and boys in their sample either in the mean age when selective mutism was first suspected or in the lag time between when it was first suspected and when it was confirmed. But we noted with interest an observation from Steinhausen and Juzi (1996) that the boys in their sample of 100 selectively mute children 'tended to start earlier with their symptoms' than the girls (at 42 months on average rather than 54 months). Was it that the symptoms started earlier or that they were noticed earlier? There is a risk that the well-justified current research interest in genetic issues and behavioural inhibition may take attention away from the sociocultural factors that can influence how and when the problem is identified. We have highlighted the possibility that such factors may play a role in the clinical referral of boys and girls both because this is an unresolved question that needs to be addressed and because each generation of researchers and clinicians ought to be aware of the possible blind spots associated with its advances in understanding.

Ethnicity and bilingualism

As noted above, the incidence of selective mutism appears to be higher in ethnic minority and immigrant groups. In their study in Birmingham primary schools Brown and Lloyd (1975) found a higher incidence of non-European families in the mute sample, in particular Afro-Caribbean families. The difference did not reach statistical significance. In a study in inner London special schools and units Cline and Kysel (1987/88) found that a relatively high proportion of the children identified by headteachers as elective mute came from ethnic minority backgrounds. Again there was some indication that Afro-Caribbean children were particularly over-represented, and again the differences did not reach statistical significance. In a study in Toronto schools Bradley and Sloman (1975) found a markedly higher incidence of elective mutism among immigrant children. These results were statistically significant (p < 0.001).

There is a good deal of support in the clinical literature for the idea that immigrant children and children from ethnic and linguistic minorities are over-represented in samples of children who are referred for selective mutism. For example, Croghan and Craven (1982) claim that 'much of the literature on elective mutism . . . is concerned with elective mute children who are bilingual'. Lesser-Katz (1986) observed that her own experience in a Spanish-speaking area in Chicago led her 'to agree that the number of silent children in immigrant communities is unusually high'. Reviewers such as Hesselman (1983) and Lebrun (1990) accepted the phenomenon as established by the 1980s, and subsequent surveys confirmed it. For example, 'immigrant' children comprised 39% of a sample of selectively mute patients in a psychiatric clinic in Zurich and 23% of a similar sample in Berlin (Steinhausen and Juzi, 1996). They commented that these figures may even underestimate the true incidence 'because immigrant families in general tend to use public mental health services less frequently than native populations' (p. 612).

The claim of minority over-representation is very difficult to test in a scientifically rigorous way. The significance of numerical data on this kind of issue can only be deduced if one knows the ethnic composition of the population from which the study sample was derived. That is not possible in this case because the clinical reports cover a wide variety of communities across developed countries. Without further population studies of selective mutism in ethnically heterogeneous areas no firm conclusion on the statistical question is possible. A more useful question to ask at this stage is whether the published case study material indicates any special features in the children from minority groups, or in their families, who are reported as selectively mute.

The first major group are children who are required at school to use a language different from the one used most often by their family at home. Generally these are children from linguistic minority backgrounds whose home language has a relatively low status in society generally. Calhoun and Koenig (1973) open their paper on elective mutism with the statement: 'Failure to speak is a fairly common referral problem according to counsellors in the Albuquerque Title 1 schools. These schools draw from lower socio-economic level families in which Spanish or an Indian language is often preferred but which is typically discouraged in the classroom.' Writing in general terms, Goll (1980) and Cline and Kysel (1987/88) highlighted the effect of the wider community's rejection of a child's first language or dialect as a language of low status. There is anecdotal evidence in some individual case histories to suggest that language status or a sense of communal rejection may have been salient for the children. Owen, a very challenging adolescent described by Youngerman (1979), was born in the USA to a woman who had come from Puerto Rico 3 years earlier. As a young boy, having learned English mainly from television, he would tease his mother for her poor command of the language. Sally (aged 8) had migrated from Canada to England and was thought by her mother a year later to be embarrassed by her strong Canadian accent (Buck, 1987). Wilma, whose family had migrated across the Atlantic in the opposite direction from Holland to Canada, confided to her brothers that she would resist speaking English (which she did successfully for a number of years) (Shaw, 1971). Even when the parents hold positions of high social status in their country of origin, children who become selectively mute often reflect tensions within the family about the use of language in their new home (Meijer, 1979, Case 2; Sluzki, 1983; Albert-Stewart, 1986). In rare cases, however, the development of selective mutism by a child in a bilingual family is seen as unrelated to the use of two languages in the home. For example, Rossouw and Lubbe (1994) thought that the use of Afrikaans and English in his home had not been a contributory factor in the pattern of speaking of 6-year-old Desmond. They argued that this was unlikely because 'these two languages are prominent in the society he lives in (white South Africa) as well as highly prominent in the media' (p. 27).

The second major group, which overlaps with the first, comprises the children of immigrant families. Most of the cases reported in the English-language literature are families from developing countries who have moved to Europe or North America. But there are also families moving between Europe and Canada (such as those mentioned in the previous paragraph) and families from the developed world moving to Africa or Asia for special reasons such as missionary work. It appears that a key factor is the process of migration as such rather than any special features of particular kinds of migration. Meijer (1979) described five cases of selective mutism seen in Israel, of whom three came from families who had recently moved between countries. He commented that anxiety, depression and loneliness are often part of the process of immigration for the parents. The capacity of the family to offer mutual support is much more seriously challenged 'because both parents need each other's support more than when alternative support figures are available and external stress is less acute'. He speculated that selective mutism may develop particularly in such families where withholding speech is an accepted way of expressing anger. One or two children in the literature had been subject to frequent moves between countries in families in which emotional support for each other was minimal (e.g. Gwen described by Pustrom and Speers, 1964). The issue of mutual emotional support in the family seems to have been a significant factor in the development of selective mutism by Lisa who was described by Atlas (1993). Her parents reacted badly after they had migrated to the USA from within an extended family network in Latin America. In what proved to be an isolated apartment in the New York metropolitan area Lisa's mother became depressed and her father isolated himself within the household. The reaction of their only child, who was 4 at the time, was to stop speaking with teachers and with family and friends when in front of other people.

The issues of migration and bilingualism often interact, as shown above. Many of the immigrant families maintain the language and customs of their country of origin in the home (e.g. a Brazilian family in Wisconsin described by Rosenbaum and Kellman, 1973). An unusual example of the impact of language isolation was the daughter of missionaries working in central Africa (Beck and Hubbard, 1987). She spoke a local African language fluently but talked English at home and with one other family close by. When this family moved away and she began to attend a French-speaking school, she ceased speaking in English to visitors, even her grandparents, and did not speak in school, although she made good progress academically. In some circumstances moving home within one's own country may have a similar effect to migration in fostering selective mutism. One example might be Jean (aged 6) who had moved five terms earlier 'from a distant part of the country where the local dialect was very different' (Sluckin, 1977).

It is almost impossible in this literature to isolate the impact of ethnic minority status *per se* from the effects of bilingualism and migration. But the themes of those describing the minority families of selectively mute children often echo the themes of the general literature on ethnicity in psychology and social work. A useful concept that was developed in the context of social work is *sociocultural dissonance*. This refers to the stress and the experience of incongruity caused by belonging to two cultures – an ethnic minority culture and the dominant culture of the society where one lives (Chau, 1989). Within the ethnic minority culture individuals often find a 'nurturing' environment that shapes their personal identity and continues to provide affective and nurturing supports. Within the institutional systems of the dominant culture they encounter a 'sustaining' environment that provides the means of survival such as goods, services, economic resources, and political power. The sustaining environment includes the institutions of the education system. Sociocultural dissonance occurs when an individual experiences incongruity because their ethnic culture conflicts in some way with the dominant culture. The key factor precipitating and maintaining the selective mutism of some of the children in ethnic minority groups may be their failure to learn how to negotiate that dissonance when they start school. For example, work with Gloria (aged 5) and her Chinese-American family convinced Meyers (1984) that 'Gloria's silence represented, in part, intense loyalty to her traditional Chinese family. She was not going to reveal any family secrets in the perceived unfriendly environment of a diverse American society.' An important element in the treatment of such children is often the participation of a member of their minority community or a speaker of their minority language who is not a member of the family, e.g. a paraprofessional from the same American Indian tribe, as described by Conrad, Delk and Williams (1974) (cf. the work with Maria described in Chapter 7 below). Goll (1980) has offered a detailed account of factors in selective mutism within 'ghetto' families. His ideas are discussed in Chapter 3.

Developmental features

Age of onset and age at referral

Early writers identified the most frequent age of reported onset as 3–5 years (e.g. Salfield, 1950). Population studies tended to confirm age of reported onset as between the age when fluent conversational speech is normally expected and the age of school entry. Initial reports are most common in the first year of kindergarten or school (e.g. Bradley and Sloman, 1975). Working in France, Myquel and Granon (1982) found two peaks for onset in a series of 14 cases. The first peak occurred at the age of 3, coinciding with entry to l'école maternelle, and the second at the age of 6 coinciding with entry to l'école primaire.

Kolvin and Fundudis (1981) emphasized the insidious development of shyness from an early age culminating in persistent selective mutism. This was clearly recorded in 19 of their series of 24 cases. Even where a more sudden late onset was described, a closer analysis of the record suggested that earlier signs of the development of the symptom had gone unrecognized at the time. Wright (1968) also reported an insidious pattern of onset in a majority of his cases, and Myquel and Granon (1982) and Steinhausen and Juzi (1996) made similar observations. In view of this insidious pattern it may be misleading to focus too confidently on a single age of onset in the majority of cases. The key factor in reported age of onset may be that a child's refusal to speak begins to impinge on adults who are concerned about such things.

Intelligence

When a child fails to speak in a key setting, such as school, investigators will often seek to exclude the possibility of mental retardation. Usually the question does not arise: the child's behaviour or speech in other settings or silent performance in that setting clearly demonstrate a good level of understanding of what is happening and a good ability to reason about events. In some early studies routine intelligence testing is reported, though intelligence level *per se* is rarely the main focus of attention in analyses of selective mutism. It is necessary to treat the reports with some caution, since the children's mutism would force examiners to depart from the standard testing procedures in many cases. However, the overall pattern of the findings is consistent, so that it is reasonable to place some reliance on them. In general the children show average to above average intelligence (e.g. 20 out of 25 cases reported by educational psychologists in one county to Buck (1987); 14 out of the 24 cases reviewed by Wright (1968); 13 out of 21 cases reviewed by Kolvin and Fundudis (1981).

On the other hand, the mean IQ reported in these studies is often below average, e.g. 83 in the series of 13 reported by Friedman and Karagan (1973) and 85 in the series of 21 reviewed by Kolvin and Fundudis (1981). Although a majority of selectively mute children are of average to good intelligence, some show moderate to severe learning difficulties. For example, a fifth of the children in the sample studied by Kolvin and Fundudis (1981) had reported non-verbal IQs below 69. There is little evidence that the development or outcome of selective mutism shows significant differences in this group. In their follow-up of 13 cases Koch and Goodlund (1973) found that the two young people who had attended classes for the educable mentally retarded were both introverted and friendless with only a limited capacity for speech ('simple replies to questions'). On the other hand, a number of individual case histories show more positive outcomes, e.g. Reed (1963); Straughan, Potter and Hamilton (1965); Ayllon and Kelly (1974); Watson (1995). In their series of 24 cases Kolvin and Fundudis (1981) found no mean IQ differences between individuals who were doing well on follow-up and those who were not.

Thus most commentators have downplayed the significance of limitations of intelligence as a factor in the development of selective mutism and in its treatment, and, in general, there has been little support for the practice of obtaining intelligence test data when children are referred for selective mutism (e.g. Hadley, 1994). But there have been thought-provoking exceptions to this consensus. Powell and Dalley (1995) argued that a formal evaluation of the mental abilities of a selectively mute

6-year-old girl enabled them to rule out 'the presence of developmental delays or mental deficiencies contributing to selective mutism' (p. 119). Klin and Volkmar (1983) reported two case studies of young people of 15 and 16 who appeared to have limited intelligence and argued that a failure to take account of this had inhibited earlier clinical interventions. On the basis of two case studies, Kristensen (1997) argued there may have been underdiagnosis of developmental problems of children with selective mutism. Subsequently this claim was supported by a substantial study of 54 children with selective mutism and 108 controls (Kristensen, 2000). In addition, a report by Russell, Raj and John (1998) describing multimodal work with children with severe learning difficulties who were selectively mute appears to demonstrate how the effectiveness of a clinical team's approach can be enhanced when children's additional learning needs are taken into account. The debate seems likely to continue on the validity and utility of intelligence assessment when clinical teams receive referrals of children with selective mutism. We will return to this issue when we discuss assessment in more detail in Chapter 7.

Speech development

A key feature in the classic definitions of selective mutism was that there is no evidence of damage to the functioning of the child's speech mechanisms, either centrally in the nervous system or peripherally in the organs used for speaking (Tramer, 1934). It remains an essential feature of contemporary definitions: as noted above, children's silence can only be described as selective if they show that they are able to speak in some settings. At the same time it has become clear that selectively mute children have a higher incidence of speech problems than is found in other groups of non-handicapped children (Kolvin and Fundudis, 1981; Wilkins, 1985). In the sample of 100 children studied by Steinhausen and Juzi (1996) over a third had a speech or language difficulty, the most common being articulation disorders (20%) and expressive language disorders (28%). Ford et al. (1998) reported similar proportions in their survey sample. When Andersson and Thomsen (1998) reviewed the hospital records of 30 selectively mute children in Denmark, they found that a third had showed delayed speech development and a further 13.5% had difficulty with articulation. There are some indications in the literature that the incidence of such problems is particularly high among those selectively mute children who are referred to speech and language therapists. Examples include unpublished papers by Carmody (1999), by Giddan et al. (1997, p. 128) and by Cleator (1998) and Wintgens (1999) which were cited by Johnson and Wintgens (2001, p. 6).

   If there is any abnormality in language comprehension or production, it is important to establish whether it (or the child's consciousness of it) could have played a significant role in causing the child's development of mutism (Rutter, 1977). For example, Meijer (1979) described a case in which a girl's slight articulation defect provoked teasing from her peers in first grade, after which she did not speak in the classroom again. Smayling (1959), who reported on five cases in which selective mutism was accompanied by speech defects, noted that the mutism decreased as her speech therapy programme progressed and the children's speech improved. Some early writers on the subject suggested that a history of mouth injury might be frequent in cases of selective mutism. Koch and Goodlund (1973) found no evidence of it in their series of 13 cases, and more recent reviewers such as Kolvin and Fundudis (1981), Tancer (1992) and Anstendig (1998) have not highlighted the issue.

It has recently been suggested that there may be differences in the development of selective mutism and its prognosis between children who have some speech and language difficulties (a 'communication disorder') and those who do not. Kristensen and Torgersen (2001) interviewed the parents of 50 selectively mute children in Norway and found that those whose children had communication disorders did not respond in the same way on a personality questionnaire as those whose children were developing speech and language normally apart from their pattern of mutism. Because most case reports have only limited data on speech and language development, it is not possible to confirm that hypothesis at this stage, but it appears to merit further research.

This chapter has focused on some basic features that define selective mutism. These features will be placed in context in Chapter 2, where we will consider the cultural meaning of the children's refusal to speak, as well as a wider range of factors within the children, their families and the community that play a part in the development of this pattern.

Chapter 2
The child, the family and the community

This chapter begins by examining cultural differences in the social meaning of speech and silence. In developed countries persistent silence in childhood is treated as rude and defiant. Children who maintain such a silence may appear shy and anxious but are often also seen as controlling and manipulative. There is great variation in when, where and to whom they are prepared to speak. Effective non-verbal communication may develop in substitution. The children are not autistic, simply not ready for the full social demands of middle childhood. In recent years a number of researchers have come to the view that anxiety plays a central role in the development and maintenance of their unusual pattern of behaviour. Some have seen selective mutism as a symptom of social phobia. These issues are discussed in the middle section of the chapter.

There has thus been increasing interest in the implications of the observation that the children appear to begin with a predisposition to problems around communication with others. Reports from clinicians and researchers working within the psychodynamic and family therapy traditions highlighted further problems in the way such predispositions are managed within the family. They frequently identified problems of communication throughout the family and particular problems within the parents' relationship. They described how a close alliance of one parent, usually the mother, with the mute child could foster strong mutual dependence that inhibited the child's social development. In places these authors appeared to lay blame on parents in a negative way, e.g. pathologizing what another observer might see as a mild example of maternal over-anxiety. In the light of more recent data on the children's genetic predispositions what was portrayed in that literature as a close alliance fostering strong mutual dependence might in fact reflect a mother's behaviour to the child she saw as most vulnerable in her family.

The families were often seen as rather isolated, so that the children did not learn about interaction with outsiders from an early age. This isolation might be particularly marked among families of selectively mute children in remote rural areas and in ethnic and linguistic minorities in urban areas. Many children were reported to develop and maintain strong relationships with peers outside the family without speaking to them. Peers, for their part, might collude with and support this use of silence.

The cultural meanings of speech and silence

Developing communication skills is central to children's socialization. Non-verbal communication skills are important, but the acquisition of speech and language is critical. Speech helps children to understand themselves and others and to communicate and validate that understanding. It enables them to express their feelings clearly to others and helps them to achieve relief from frustration and stress. It is a basic tool in the move towards mastery of the environment, independence and maturity. Ultimately the way a person speaks and the vocabulary they use become important expressions of their personal identity.

Silence is a counterpart of speech with its own conventions that mirror those of speech. A child must learn to talk and must also learn when not to talk, including how to conduct oneself in silence. Keeping silent in the company of others, like speaking to them, is an act of communication. Through posture and gesture, and through the use of the eyes and facial expression, silence in particular contexts in the English-speaking world may communicate assent, boredom, puzzlement, respect, resistance, overwhelming sadness . . . a range of possibilities. Silence may have a particular significance in formal rituals. In different cultures, according to the setting, convention may take it to denote acquiescence or refusal, questioning or command, warning or insult. Some commentators on selective mutism have emphasized that the phenomenon cannot be fully understood without considering the uses and significance of silence in communication. Hadley (1994) argued that it is necessary to 'address the healthy manifestations of silence . . . healthy silence user roles . . . and with it the wider meaning of speech refusal' (p. xxii).

The old English adage 'speech is silvern but silence is golden' derived from religious sentiment. Zeligs (1961) traces it back to rabbinical commentaries in early Jewish literature: 'If a word is worth one selah, silence is worth two. (Silence invokes Thy praise.)' He points out that this advice was secularized in later Hebrew tradition: there is a potential material advantage in keeping one's own counsel. Similar sentiments are expressed in proverbs in other languages, such as 'because of the mouth the fish dies' (Spanish) and 'man becomes wise through the ear' (Farsi) (Saville-Troike, 1982). In many cultures silence is associated with strength – with greater knowledge and greater potential for action than one cares to claim aloud. In modern North America and elsewhere the hero is often portrayed as a 'strong, silent man'. In some traditional cultures, such as that of the Burundi as described by Albert (1964), the silence of a person of high rank can prevent others speaking.

The emphasis on speech in socialization may be a particular character-istic of our highly verbal and individualistic culture. 'One only has to be silent for a few moments before one hears people ask, "What's wrong?"' (Hadley, 1994, p. xxiii). There are many cultures in which it is quite nor-mal for a conversation to include periods of silence that would be a source of embarrassment in a conversation between English-speaking people. For, example, if Western Apache in the recent past found them-selves in a social situation where there was an element of uncertainty or unpredictability, the most appropriate response was silence (Basso, 1970). It has been reported that the Paliyans of South India communicate very little at all times and become 'almost silent by the age of 40' (Gardner, 1966, quoted by Saville-Troike, 1982). Perhaps selective mutism is mainly a problem of modern developed countries. In many cultures the children's behaviour would not appear puzzling or problematic in the same way. In many settings across the world and over time it would have been expected that children would remain silent outside the circle of a very small group of intimates. In some cultures children have been taught that they may speak freely with other children (and perhaps with servants or adults of lower social status) but must be 'seen and not heard' in the presence of their parents and of adults in their social circle.

The structures underpinning socialization in Western society may even exacerbate the problem: it is no accident that the main source of referrals of selectively mute children are schools. In Chapter 4 the social functions of schooling in isolated communities are discussed in more detail, and an example is given of a community in which the building of new schools far-ther from children's home communities appeared to lead to an increased incidence of selective mutism. Saville-Troike (1982) has argued that 'the relative silence of some children (e.g. Chinese, Japanese, and Hopi) over others (e.g. British and American) may be related to childrearing practices and values regarding the relative value of individual achievements and ini-tiative: children in societies which value individual achievement generally talk more'. She also suggested that in those cultures in which children tend to be less verbal about their needs and wishes their early experience seems to include closer physical contact with their caretakers. Within such cultures there is an expectation that adults or older siblings will care for young children without need for verbalization. 'This also relates to atti-tudes even in the adult speech community that people should not, and should not have to, ask directly for what they want' (p. 227).

The literature on selective mutism is full of moralistic and negative comment. Adults in developed countries expect to meet the dependency needs of children and tend to feel impotent to do so when they will not communicate. An inability to communicate (e.g. because of handicap) is experienced as a challenge; a refusal to communicate can seem to repre-sent a wilful defiance and a threat. In correspondence teachers have commented: 'I felt it was a failure on my part and I did get annoyed'; 'I was to feel very disappointed and at a loss when she would not speak';

'Sarah's failure to talk embarrassed adults. Her mother thought she appeared 'ignorant''. Chethik (1975) acknowledged the 'intense emotional wear and tear' that a child's persistent silence creates for a psychotherapist, and Subak, West and Carlin (1982) wrote of 'a sense of failure . . . ensuing anger and the challenge to the therapist's sense of competence'. Ruzicka and Sackin (1974) described therapists' 'painful feelings of helplessness, worthlessness, frustration and rage'. Over-reaction by the authorities is common: approximately half of the 13 children reviewed by Friedman and Karagan (1973) had been threatened with dismissal from school because of their refusal to talk.

The child

Behavioural inhibition

Early studies of selective mutism often mentioned temperamental characteristics such as shyness which will be discussed later in this section. But the early investigators did not have a satisfactory framework of developmental theory that they could apply to their observations. Re-reading some of their reports suggests that some children who later develop selective mutism show behavioural inhibition in their first two years. In order to provide a context for later discussion in the book, we begin this account of the children with a summary of recent developments in the understanding of behavioural inhibition. For a full review see Oosterlaan (2001).

The temperamental characteristic of inhibition has been defined as a 'temperamentally-based predisposition to react consistently to novel and unfamiliar events, both social and non-social, with initial restraint and avoidance together with signs of wariness and fear' (Reznick et al., 1992 quoted by Oosterlaan, 2001, pp. 45–46). The major longitudinal studies that laid the basis for recent thinking on the subject were undertaken by Kagan, Reznick and Snidman (1987). They demonstrated that in young children there was a correlation between some physiological characteristics, in particular differences in the threshold of reactivity in parts of the limbic system, and behavioural reactions to unfamiliar and challenging events. They followed up two groups of young children, selected at either 21 or 30 months from larger groups, because they showed markedly inhibited or uninhibited behaviour when they were exposed to unfamiliar rooms, people and events. The first group were followed up at 4 and at 5 years, and the second group at 3 and 5 years. The indices of behavioural inhibition in the younger group were long delays in interacting with, or immediate retreat from, unfamiliar people or objects, ceasing to play or vocalize, and seeking proximity to the mother after temporary separation. Similar signs of inhibition were seen in the older group for whom the index of inhibited behaviour was based on the children's behaviour with an unfamiliar child of the same age and sex, and on behaviour with an unfamiliar woman.The researchers examined a range of physiological signs such as heart rate, dilatation of pupils, muscle tension and biochemical indicators of neurotransmitter activity. Measurement of eight separate physiological variables showed that the inhibited children were more likely to show the physiological signs that would be predicted from lower thresholds of reactivity. There was a high correlation between the aggregate mean of all eight physiological variables taken at 5 years with the index of behavioural inhibition at 21 months and a lower but still statistically significant correlation with behavioural inhibition measures taken when the children were older. The follow-up studies also showed that the children's patterns of inhibited or uninhibited behaviour remained significantly stable over time.

It is relevant to this book that one of the most sensitive indices of inhibition at 5 years was the inhibited children's reluctance to talk spontaneously to the examiner, in contrast to the uninhibited children. There is some empirical support for the suggestion that behavioural inhibition may predispose children to develop anxiety disorders, in particular children who remain consistently inhibited over time and children who have parents with anxiety disorders. However, after reviewing the evidence Oosterlaan (2001) highlighted some important methodological concerns which may reduce the generalizability of the studies on which this conclusion relies. Firstly, most of the studies used the same two groups of participants in the USA who were followed up by Kagan and his colleagues over an extended period. (The one exception was a study by Caspi, Elder and Bem (1996) who carried out an 18-year follow-up of a group of children in Dunedin, New Zealand.) Secondly, the studies differed in the time window in which the rates of anxiety disorders were assessed. Thus the case for a link between behavioural inhibition in infancy and the later development of anxiety disorders can be regarded as only partially proven.

There is evidence that two temperamental characteristics associated with behavioural inhibition are relatively common in selectively mute children. Ford et al. (1998) reported that those featured in their survey typically did not respond well to novel stimuli and did not handle transitions and change well. In a study by Black and Uhde (1995) 90% of the selectively mute children met the diagnostic criteria for 'avoidant disorder'. The possible role of behavioural inhibition in the development of selective mutism will be discussed more fully in the next chapter.

Anxiety and passivity

The most prominent characteristics of the majority of selectively mute children are anxiety and timidity. In different samples Steinhausen and Juzi (1996) and Ford et al. (1998) found that selectively mute children obtained higher scores for internalized problems than for externalized problems on a standard questionnaire, the Child Behavior Checklist. Of the clinical sample of 100 children studied by Steinhausen and Juzi

(1996) 85% were described as shy and 66% as anxious. In recent years there has been increasing support for the view that, although many factors may play a part in the development of selective mutism, anxiety should be recognized as 'the underlying driving force of the disorder' (Donnelly, 1998, p. 224). It is argued that, when the children are manipulative or controlling in their behaviour, 'it is more helpful and accurate to view the mutism as an involuntary defence against the child's severe anxiety' (Anstendig, 1998, p. 429). Among the arguments given in support of this opinion are:

- The majority of the selectively mute children seen at some centres, such as the National Institute of Mental Health in the USA, appeared shy and and anxious rather than oppositional or negative (Leonard and Topol, 1993, p. 697). Some area surveys and follow-up studies have confirmed this finding (Black and Uhde, 1995; Steinhausen and Juzi, 1996; Dummit et al., 1997).
- It is often reported that other family members show shyness or high levels of anxiety, and there is evidence that these characteristics may have a genetic basis (Leonard and Topol, 1993; Black and Uhde, 1995; Leonard and Dow, 1995; Kristensen and Torgersen, 2001).
- Some selectively mute children are rather inactive and passive, tending to be inhibited in all their behaviour, which is seen as suggestive of an underlying heightened level of anxiety (Anstendig, 1998).
- When children have associated problems in addition to their mutism, they tend to be anxiety-related problems such as social phobia (see below) rather than motivational or conduct problems (Black and Uhde, 1995).
- Some drugs that are successful in the treatment of anxiety disorders have been found to be effective in the treatment of selective mutism as well (see Chapter 8).

These are compelling arguments, and it is no longer possible to ignore the central role of anxiety in selective mutism. However, attributing a central role to anxiety does not mean that other factors play no part and, if there are oppositional and manipulative tendencies in a child's behaviour, they cannot be ignored when planning intervention. We consider that in all cases of selective mutism it is necessary to investigate both issues of anxiety and issues of control: the safe working assumption in the initial stages of assessment will be that difficulties exist in both areas.

Selective mutism as a symptom of social phobia

Social phobia involves 'a marked and persistent fear of one or more social or performance situations in which the person is exposed to unfamiliar people or to possible scrutiny by others. The individual fears that he or she will act in a way (or show anxiety symptoms) that will be humiliating or embarrassing' (APA, 1994, p. 416). Sufferers experience intense anxiety, even to the point of a panic attack, on exposure to situations of that kind. They may have specific fears about performing certain activities, such as writing, eating, or speaking in front of others, or they may simply have a vague, non-specific general fear of embarrassing themselves. Many children and adolescents show some social anxiety or self-consciousness, but extreme anxiety of this kind that interferes with a child's ability to function is not common.

Some children with selective mutism show signs of social phobia, and its symptoms in a mild or severe form are often reported in family members. When animals face a threatening situation, they are often quiet and withdrawn. That is also how young children behave when they feel anxious on meeting strangers. Lesser-Katz (1986), Black and Uhde (1992) and others have argued that selective mutism may grow out of stranger anxiety and may be better thought of as 'a manifestation of social phobia rather than a separate diagnostic entity' (p. 1093). If that is the case, they suggested, an appropriate diagnosis might help to determine what form of treatment would be most effective. One source of support for this position is a finding that as many as 8% of a sample of 7–13-year-olds who had been diagnosed with social phobia also presented symptoms of selective mutism (Beidel, Turner and Morris, 1999).When Crumley (1990) asked a young adult who had been selectively mute as a child to recall his experiences, his memory was of intense panic attacks when called upon to talk. Crumley saw this as suggestive of social phobia (cf. Crumley, 1993).

However, there are problems with an over-simple statement of the position. It is difficult to see how selective mutism can be an expression of or a result of social phobia when most commentators see social phobia as developing rather later in childhood than is usual with selective mutism. One survey suggested that the average age of onset of social phobia is between 11.3 and 12.3 years (Last et al., 1992). This could be because self-consciousness is a central prerequisite for the development of social phobia.

> The abilities to see oneself as a social object and to experience embarrassment may emerge around age 4 or 5 years (Buss, Iscoe and Puss, 1979), whereas the abilities to take others' perspectives and then to anticipate and feel clear concern over negative evaluation from others probably do not fully develop until around 8 years of age . . . Thus, by late childhood and early adolescence, social and evaluation fears are forefront. Social phobia is thought to evolve from normal anxiety that is magnified by the social demands of preadolescence. (Velting and Albino, 2001, p. 128)

Thus the developmental patterns of selective mutism and social phobia make it impossible to think of the former as an outcome or 'manifestation' of the latter. However, that does not undermine the more common view that the two are 'closely related' (Pine and Grun, 1998, p. 119).

Among reviewers espousing this view is Anstendig (1999). The arguments in support include evidence that:

- Both occur more commonly in girls than in boys (see Chapter 1).
- Both are often associated with the temperamental characteristic of 'behavioural inhibition' (for social phobia, for example, see Hayward et al., 1998).
- Both appear to have a genetic basis as they occur more often when other family members show shyness or other similar patterns of behaviour (see below).
- There is some evidence that they can be treated with the same forms of medication. Beidel and Randall (1994, p. 121) cited the examples of phenelzine and fluoxetine. (For a discussion of drug therapy for selective mutism, see Chapter 8.)
- Those who have had selective mutism and overcome it, often continue to report that they find difficulty conversing and feel uncomfortable in social situations – 'not unlike characteristics found in social phobia' (Ford et al., 1998, p. 203).

Putting together this kind of evidence and the evidence of 'a marked desynchronicity between the apparent ages of onset for the two disorders', Bergman, Piacentini and McCracken (2002) suggested that selective mutism may be 'a developmental subtype of SP [social phobia] with earlier onset than other symptoms of the disorder' (p. 939). They pointed out that there is some anecdotal evidence that adults who were affected by selective mutism as children may continue to suffer from social anxiety in later life. Issues relating to follow-up research will be discussed in the final chapter of this book.

Controlling behaviour

After reading an article on selective mutism in a daily newspaper a young woman wrote to the author recalling her experience of it as a child:

> My unwillingness to speak didn't bother me too much. I was never upset by it or felt odd. The fact was I was odd, and I sometimes wonder whether I sometimes relished it. I was taken to a child psychiatrist but to no avail. When I was 7, one of my teachers implored me just to whisper to her alone, or to just start by whispering to my best friend (how I had friends I can't imagine). However, I refused to give in. As time wore on I became more and more resilient. I hated the teachers pestering me and saw them rather as the enemy.

The children may be shy, timid and fearful in some contexts, and anxiety may be an underlying factor in many, or even most, cases, but those who come to know the children well, such as the teachers whose accounts were quoted in Chapter 1, also remark on something else. They observe that a refusal to speak can gain control for a child over an aspect of the social world that is normally dominated by adults. In reviewing 24 cases Wright (1968) observed that each record referred to controlling behaviour at some point and that the parents generally reported the children to be strong-willed and difficult to manage at home. He emphasized 'an excessive need to control' as one of the central features of selective mutism. These features are then carried over into the children's relationships with teachers and others in their environment. Some surveys have suggested that this is very common. For example, it was reported in 18 out of 20 cases seen at one centre in the USA (Krohn, Weckstein and Wright, 1992).

Other surveys, however, have indicated a much lower incidence of controlling behaviour (Black and Uhde, 1995; Steinhausen and Juzi, 1996). Shyness and anxiety appear to be characteristic of a much higher proportion of those studied across samples. It may be that the impact of controlling behaviour was over-emphasized in some early reports because it had not been expected. There are good reasons for thinking that some manipulative and demanding behaviour is triggered by anxiety that the child cannot control. At times it may possibly also be a reaction to repeated efforts to make them speak.

As a result the literature has some extreme examples of controlling behaviour going beyond the refusal to speak: in one of Wright's cases the parents changed the name of a younger sibling at the selectively mute child's insistence; in another the child succeeded in insisting that her mother cook entirely different meals for her from the rest of the family; a 7-year-old in the series described by Goll (1980) insisted on being held like a baby when answering the call of nature and always slept with his clothes on because he simply refused to change at bedtime (p. 147). However, the most effective control strategy for most of the children centres on the refusal of speech. They are often remarkably successful in achieving compliance by others in elaborate arrangements to get round their silence.

Reed (1963) introduced the influential notion that selectively mute children can be categorized into two distinct groups – one comprising those who are comparatively relaxed but unresponsive, negativistic and manipulative, and the other comprising those who are tense and anxious, associating speech with fear. A number of clinical investigators have highlighted these two patterns in the children they have seen. For example, Koch and Goodlund (1973) reviewed the records of 13 cases and found that 61% had shown shyness and 54% rebelliousness at the time of referral. In a preschool programme Lesser-Katz (1986) studied 15 selectively mute children and found that 12 of them were shy and reticent: 'If asked to sit, stand or walk, they would comply – but woodenly.' The other three children were not compliant but rather resistant and 'oppositional'. They 'refused to participate in any activities suggested by their teachers or any other adult, opting to do things on their own . . . [and maintaining] a physical distance which they jealously controlled'.

Such analyses seem to support Reed's notion of two major subtypes of selective mutism. However, Kolvin and Fundudis (1981) reviewing 24 cases found a more complex picture. They identified '. . . almost invariably a streak of negativism and poor malleability both at school and at home'. Half the children presented as 'rather sulky to strangers and rather aggressive at home. About one quarter combined shyness in social situations with an apparently submissive attitude in the home, and the other quarter seemed to be very sensitive children who tended to weep and be easily distressed either in social or home situations'. The distinction Reed drew between a pattern of shyness and an oppositional pattern is of some value, but there are dangers in placing too much reliance on it. Reed himself based it on a study of just four cases. In practice few children can be categorized simplistically as *either* anxious *or* manipulative. Wright (1968) observed that in his sample even children who presented as shy and anxious in some situations were often found to be obstinate and controlling in others. Lesser-Katz (1986) described the resistant behaviour of three children in her sample as a 'fight response to fear'. On the other hand, Croghan and Craven (1982) also emphasized the importance of recognizing the anxiety associated with speaking even in a child who presents as attention-seeking and manipulative. Their interventions with JB over 18 months were ineffective until they took account of this point. In another case a child's overwhelming anxiety about being on her own with the therapist in play therapy sessions led her to scream or regress in each one until her mother was invited to join her from the fifth session. She then calmed down and was able to use the opportunity so that these sessions could complement other school-based interventions (Afnan and Carr, 1989). (The work with this child, Jenny, is described in more detail in Chapters 5 and 7.)

Patterns of communication

There is great variety in the patterns of selective communication that the children show in their everyday behaviour. For each individual it is necessary to ask, who do they talk to? in what manner? how often? under what conditions? what is their non-verbal behaviour in different situations? These questions have often been the subject of comment but have only been investigated in a systematic way in recent years. In one survey a large group of respondents rated the situations that most affected how often a person with selective mutism talked as being with strangers, at school, in social events, in new settings, in family gatherings and when there was some degree of stress or anxiety (Ford et al., 1998). The pattern of talking and not talking can be highly complex. For example, children may select only one family member to speak to and may restrict themselves to whispering even then (Austad, Sininger and Stricken, 1980) or may speak to peers outside the home only when no adults are within hearing (Wright et al., 1985, p. 741). Adults are often impressed, even a little intimidated, by the consistent way in which children keep to their 'rules'. Smayling (1959) described a boy aged 10 who was an outstanding player on the class baseball team. His mutism did not permit 'the slightest grunt or gasp upon his catching, throwing, hitting or missing a particularly fast ball'. Johnson and Wintgens (2001) described a child who 'broke her arm at playtime but did not tell anyone until she got home' (p. 21).

Many reports highlight a marked contrast: children who stay silent in some settings communicate very easily in others. They may, for example, use the telephone to talk to people with whom they would not converse in person (Browne, Wilson and Laybourne, 1963). In some cases children are even seen as talking too much, at least at home (Sluckin, 1977; Crema and Kerr, 1978).

> It was almost as though we (mother and teacher) were talking about two different children, one at home and one at school, because Mrs P. said that at home Anita could be bossy with her younger sister, then aged 2, and rude and defiant towards her parents, whereas at school she seemed inhibited and conforming. Her mother did say, though, that Anita could be shy with people she did not know . . . [She] was extremely talkative at home, so talkative in fact that she had to be told to be quiet at times. Her mother wished that the talking could be shared out between home and school! Apparently, when Anita was not talking to other people, she was talking to herself.
>
> Teacher, 1985

In a very small number of cases children have been reported to be mute at home rather than elsewhere (Wilkins, 1985; Szabo, 1996). These children generally show an unusual pattern of development so that their selective mutism appears to have different roots from that of most of the children discussed in this book. Two of the three young people described by Wilkins (1985) were in early adolescence, and their refusal to speak at home seemed to be a direct reaction to family difficulties. The mutism described by Szabo (1996) was also a reaction to family behaviour (see Chapter 1).

A rather larger number of reports describe a pattern in which the child is mute outside the home and also inhibited or selective in speaking within the family. For example, William (aged 10), who had never to anyone's knowledge spoken a word outside or at school, spoke only infrequently at home and then just to one older brother (he was the seventh of eight children) (Bednar, 1974). Mary (aged 9) avoided her father whenever possible and communicated with him only through her mother. 'The only persons with whom Mary could be reasonably relaxed and uninhibited were her brother, one year her senior, and a 6-year-old girl who lived in the neighborhood. With these two children Mary played enthusiastically, spoke freely, and sometimes even laughed openly' (Ruzicka and Sackin, 1974). One child who had experienced multiple changes of carer was selectively mute within the home but proved to be unusually ready to speak to the clinician working with him – once his uncle and new step-mother had left the room (Louden, 1987).

Even in settings in which they do not speak at all, some selectively mute children do not appear socially isolated. The lack of speech does not prevent them from communicating non-verbally with others. Reports exist of an impressive variety of strategies for doing so: smiling, nodding, head-shaking and shrugging (Bednar, 1974; Albert-Stewart, 1986); girlish giggling, writing messages on a pad, and using a guttural or snorting sound to accompany gestures (Ambrosino and Alessi, 1979); tapping in rhythmic dialogue (Heimlich, 1981); tapping a teacher's shoulder to gain attention and then miming what he needs (report from teacher, 1986). In fact selectively mute children often receive constant positive reinforcement for effective non-verbal communication – perhaps to the point where they are released from any pressure to speak (Van der Kooy and Webster, 1975).

This picture of seemingly lively substitutes for speaking cannot be over-generalized. LeRoy (aged 6) did not begin to smile at school until he began to talk (Strait, 1958). Some of the children show a general passive immobility (Parker, Olsen and Throckmorton 1960), minimal eye contact and 'severe behavioral constriction with strangers' (Rosenberg and Lindblad, 1978), a lack of facial expression and tightly sealed lips (Scott, 1977), or a face like a mask (Chethik, 1975; Buck, 1987). The child presents as 'a pliable mannequin' (Wulbert et al., 1973). Posture may be tense and stiff (Hayden, 1980; Hesselman, 1983; Lesser-Katz, 1986), and a child may move slowly and lethargically in some settings (Ciottone and Madonna, 1984). In extreme cases children may be unable to form some movements when attention is focused on them (Hill and Scull, 1985) or even unable to walk without assistance (Roberts, 1984). Typically, as speech improves and generalizes, the children's posture relaxes and gestures appear that were not in their repertoire before (Tittnich, 1990). Strait (1958) quoted LeRoy's teacher as saying at this stage: 'He beams'.

When selectively mute, the apparent passivity of the children's stance is often belied by their alert watchfulness, an intense concentration on the activities and communications of others that amounts to an active show of interest. The conflict they experience about communication is vividly portrayed in an account of the behaviour of John (aged 12) shortly after admission to an inpatient hospital ward. Wassing (1973) explains:

> . . . he remained completely silent right from the start. In the beginning he also kept himself fully in the background. He did not mix with the others, neither with his peers nor with any of the group workers. He stayed passive, restricting himself to watching the actions of the others around him. After a while, however, he gave up his isolation a little bit and he started to approach his group members. He would post himself quite near them, showing an expression on his face that seemed to disclose an eagerness to join in their activities. But he typically could not induce himself to make any

further moves to bring this desire to effect. He would merely stand very close to the others, with tight lips and in a rigid posture, only signalling through the medium of his eyes, which expressed a keen expectation, that he wanted to participate. By not uttering one word he demonstrated an impotence to make the step that, in the given social context, would have been the appropriate one for him to make. While thus manifesting an inability to accommodate to the obvious expectations of his peers, he on the other hand, by his very attitude, seemed to send the message that he, on his part, expected the others to accommodate to him instead, by taking over the initiative from him.

A number of clinicians and investigators have suggested ways of categorizing the stages between complete silence and normal conversational talking in the patterns of communication of selectively mute children. A well-structured example was outlined by Johnson and Wintgens (2001, p. 69); see Table 2.1. Some observers would suggest variants on stages 5–7 of that list, emphasizing the significance of children whispering, talking with less volume and talking with less spontaneity than is usual (e.g. Ford et al., 1998, p. 206).

Table 2.1 Stages of confident speaking

1	Does not communicate nor participate
2	Cooperates but limited communication
3	Communicates through visual, non-verbal means
4	Uses non-verbal sounds
5	Speaks within earshot of person but not directly to them
6	Uses single words with selected people
7	Uses connected speech with selected people
8	Begins to generalize to a range of people
9	Begins to generalize to a range of settings
10	Communicates freely

Source: Johnson and Wintgens (2001), p. 69.

Associated characteristics and behaviour

Selectively mute children are a heterogeneous group, but some associated personality characteristics are commonly found alongside the pattern of a selective withdrawal of speech. Anxiety, shyness and obstinacy have been discussed above. Other features that regularly appear in accounts of the children are social immaturity, hypersensitivity, aggressiveness and temper tantrums. Reviewing five cases Meijer (1979) wrote of 'a rather developed sense of vulnerability to being hurt or of being left without essential protection and support'. Many of the children show intense specific fears that are controlled in some cases by elaborate rituals. For example, Amy (aged 6) was afraid of dogs to the point that she would sometimes avoid going out in the street, was afraid of being alone, and was always fearful at bedtime, going through a series of procedures before she could stay in bed (Chethik, 1975). (Cf. Pustrom and Speers, 1964, p. 289; Hayden, 1983, p. 16.) Some clinicians have interpreted this kind of concern for protective rituals as a co-morbid obsessive–compulsive disorder (e.g. Leonard and Topol, 1993). But in most case studies where the relevant material is described in detail, a combination of anxiety and behavioural inhibition underlying selective mutism seems sufficient to explain the pattern of ritualistic behaviour without invoking a further diagnostic label.

Some early investigators suggested that a child's fear of speaking might arise from a trauma associated with the mouth such as an injury or frightening dental treatment. Parker, Olsen and Throckmorton MC (1960), who espoused this view, were able to present only the weakest evidence for it (p. 66). Survey evidence does not support the suggestion (Black and Uhde, 1995). There are many more reports of selectively mute children with specific fears that do not have a direct connection with speech or the mouth.

In the past it was frequently reported that selectively mute children have enuresis or encopresis. A problem of this kind featured in 46% of the cases reviewed by Kolvin and Fundudis (1981), in a similar proportion of the smaller numbers of cases reviewed by Pustrom and Speers (1964) and Schachter (1981), and in very many of the individual case studies in the literature. More recent surveys, however, have sometimes indicated a lower rate of incidence: only one of the 24 cases reviewed by Wilkins (1985) had nocturnal enuresis and only two of the 50 cases surveyed by Dummit et al. (1997). These figures seem very low, however, and some recent surveys offer midway estimates: 25% of the sample of 100 children with selective mutism studied by Steinhausen and Juzi (1996) were reported to have had a history of the problem, and nearly one third of the children studied by Kristensen (2000). Black and Uhde (1995), who found that 17% of the 30 children they surveyed had a history of enuresis, pointed out that this figure is 'not much different from that found in previous studies of the general population' (p. 853).

The wide variation in the incidence of enuresis reported by clinicians may reflect different levels of interest in the symptom at the point when a history is taken. Psychodynamic commentators highlighted developmental links between problems of speech acquisition and problems of toilet training (e.g. Youngerman, 1979). Writers in the behavioural tradition pointed to similar contingencies affecting both functions and highlighted situations in which children's reluctance to speak has the consequence of them failing to warn that they need to use the toilet (e.g. Wright et al.,1985, p. 741). Sometimes wetting seems to have been associated with the children's underlying determination to have others take responsibility for their care and protection. For example, Amy (aged 5) would 'wet her pants at school if the teachers forgot to ask her if she needed to go to the bathroom, although she had been told that she could go to the bathroom anytime' (Barlow, Strother and Landreth, 1986). (Current concerns about fire safety in schools sometimes lead to a rule that children are not allowed to leave their classroom without asking, even to go to the toilet. In schools with such rules a teacher may accommodate the needs of a selectively mute pupil by agreeing on a non-verbal signal.)

It may be imagined that going to school will be an unpleasant experience for many of the children. School phobia, generally in mild form, has been reported on occasions (e.g. Elson et al., 1965; Subak, West and Carlin, 1982), but it does not feature prominently in the literature and is not reported as a problem associated with selective mutism in any recent survey (Steinhausen and Juzi, 1996; Ford et al., 1998; Kristensen, 2000). In fact, a remarkable characteristic of the overall picture is that the children rarely refuse to go to school. They therefore appear to show a dogged determination not only in maintaining their silence but also in allowing themselves to be placed regularly in situations in which their social withdrawal is challenged and exposed.

The family

In this section of the chapter we draw extensively on early case studies, partly because more recent reports in the behavioural tradition have tended to ignore family dynamics in selective mutism. The outline picture that is presented here may have been influenced by clinicians' readiness to pathologize families and by difficulties some family members experienced in communicating their feelings in a clinic setting. Recent psychiatric surveys of larger groups of selective mute children and their families, such as that of Steinhausen and Juzi (1996), have tended to ignore issues of family dynamics in favour of the analysis of diagnostic categories and co-morbidity. Where relevant survey evidence is available, it is cited in the text below. But readers should note that, in general, that evidence is sparse, and this section remains, as it was in the first edition of the book, excessively reliant on judgments formed by early clinical investigators.

Speech patterns in the children's families

Selectively mute children often come from families who would be described by their neighbours as very quiet. There is often a family history of shyness at the least and even of some childhood mutism. In Tramer's classic account of an 8-year-old boy who was selectively mute, his mother and all of his five siblings were described as having been very shy from their early days (Tramer, 1934). In another early report Salfield (1950) mentions that the grandfather of William (aged 7) who lived in the same rural area would go about for prolonged periods without speaking. 'He will, for instance, go into the village post-office-cum-general-store, thrust half a crown under the grille, speechless, and when given in exchange the wrong thing, he just pushes it back and waits for the next offer, till finally the purchase is completed to his satisfaction.' Similarly, John (aged 7), who was described by Buck (1987), had a paternal aunt with a history of rarely speaking at school.

Brown and Lloyd (1975) found that either one or both parents of half the selectively mute children in their survey were described as shy whereas only about 7% of the parents of control children were in this category. Shyness and reserve were noted in 9 of the 11 families of selectively mute children studied by Wergeland (1979). In a clinical sample Steinhausen and Adamek (1997) found that first-, second- and third-degree relatives of children with selective mutism were three times as likely to be reported to be taciturn as those of children seen in the same institution for other emotional and communication problems. In a survey by Black and Uhde (1995) over a third of the households had a history of selective mutism in the immediate family. Kristensen (2000) found a lower rate of one fifth, and Steinhausen and Adamek found a much lower proportion (e.g. 8% of mothers), but this figure was still well above the rate for their control group.

The observation that the parents see themselves as relatively quiet people is often a feature of the individual case study reports (e.g. Friedman and Karagan, 1973; Colligan, Colligan and Dillard, 1977; Sluckin, 1977, Case 1). It is not uncommon for shy or mute behaviour to be prevalent throughout the family. One example is the family of Linda (aged 6) who had never spoken, to anyone's knowledge, outside her immediate family circle (Scott, 1977). Both her mother and her maternal grandmother had been extremely shy as children. One of her brothers found it difficult to separate from the family when he first started school, and her other brother and her sister both took a year in school before they began communicating with their teacher.

Where there is a family history of this kind, it is likely that there is a genetically transmitted temperamental predisposition towards shyness. In addition, it is likely that an important factor in the development of the child's mute stance will be social learning within the family. This has never been studied directly, but reported observations suggest various ways in which the process may work. Parents' behaviours that are seen as supporting the development of normal communication patterns include:

- When the child starts speaking, both parents expect/demand speech in everyday situations, including contacts with people who are unfamiliar.
- Both parents model relaxed verbal communication with others.
- Both parents are open in their own conversations with others and relaxed about what their children may say to others.

In contrast, parents' behaviours that are seen as supporting the development of selective mutism include:

- When the child starts speaking, one or both parents do not hold out an expectation that the child will talk to others in everyday situations, especially if they are unfamiliar.

- One or both parents do not speak easily with visitors to the home or people outside the household.
- One or both parents are very cautious about some topics in conversation and place restrictions on what their children should talk about with others.

In early case studies it was sometimes suggested that a key factor in the child's development of reticence or mutism was not direct modelling or suggestion but disturbing or distorted messages about speaking that are conveyed by parents and others. In a number of case reports in the literature there is a record of family concern about the disclosure of family secrets to people outside the family circle (e.g. Looff, 1971; Wergeland, 1979). Working in an inner city area Lesser-Katz (1986) highlighted the situation of households dependent on state assistance where it was important that fathers' occasional earnings from odd jobs should be kept secret. In a rural area Looff (1971) highlighted a mother's sense of shame about her husband's drinking bouts in the face of church disapproval. Pustrom and Speers (1964) illustrated the convoluted way in which such concerns might be expressed. Bobby (aged 8) had a paternal grandmother who was receiving psychiatric treatment. The children were repeatedly cautioned not to talk to her for fear they might divulge family secrets from the parents' rows which she, in her turn, would tell the psychiatrist (cf. Case 2 in the same report). However the taboo on disclosure was expressed, the effect for the selectively mute child was seen to be the same – to reinforce a sense that it is good to stay silent with those outside the home.

In extreme cases the pattern of selective mutism has sometimes appeared to be associated with child abuse – a little-understood association that requires further research (Adams and Glasner, 1954; Hayden, 1980, p. 125; Hayden, 1983). Great care is required in interpreting material in this field. There have been isolated case reports in which a selectively mute child is shown to have had a history of physical or sexual abuse (e.g. Jacobsen, 1995). But some commentary which has highlighted the issue has cited case reports in which a child was related to a victim of violence but had not themselves been a direct victim (e.g. Maskey, 2001 citing Szabo, 1996). If claims of an association are taken at their face value, it could lead to professionals believing that selective mutism should be taken as a possible symptom of abuse so that a referral of the former should lead to an investigation to check for the latter (Leonard and Topol, 1993).

The basis for that judgement might be findings such as that of Black and Uhde (1995) who observed that parents of four of the thirty selectively mute children whom they studied (13%) reported a history of physical or sexual abuse. They commented, however:

> Two of these subjects had onset of SM before suffering a single incident of sexual abuse by a non-family member. Another child suffered chronic mild abuse and neglect by his mother from age 2 until she abandoned the

family when he was 4½ years old. He was subsequently well cared for by his father. Age of onset of SM was unclear, but it was at approximately age 4 or 5. One boy was briefly mistreated by his father at 18 months of age. The father was sent to prison for sexually abusing an older sister shortly there-after. There was no clear temporal or causal relationship between the onset of SM and the abuse in any case. (pp. 851–852)

In a larger survey involving 153 families Ford et al. (1998) found that 2% identified physical abuse as a precipitating cause of selective mutism and 1.3% identified sexual abuse. McGregor, Pullar and Cundall (1994) carried out a retrospective case-control study of children identified by schools as selectively mute in one English city. They examined school medical records, the child protection database held by community paedi-atric departments and the child protection register held by the social services department. They found evidence of definite or probable abuse in 8 out of 18 case records relating to children with selective mutism com-pared with only one amongst two groups of controls. There are methodological reasons for treating the data with caution: children iden-tified as selectively mute may have been more likely than controls to be investigated for possible family abuse, and headteachers' recall of ex-pupils with selective mutism may have been more vivid in cases where an additional factor such as suspected abuse has played a part in the history. The authors confidently drew the conclusion that 'many types of trau-matic experience may precipitate elective mutism, but it is likely that child abuse, particularly child sexual abuse, is a causal factor in some subjects' (p. 541). However, further studies are required to support that conclu-sion, when other group studies have yielded such different findings. The question of a possible association between experience of abuse and the development of selective mutism remains open. Neither clinical reports nor survey data have yet satisfactorily resolved it. There is no basis from the available evidence for treating selective mutism as a probable indica-tor that a child has been abused.

Family characteristics and structure

When Wilkins (1985) compared 24 selectively mute children in a clinic sample with 24 children referred for other emotional disorders he found that the families of the former were intact much more often than was the case with the controls. All the selectively mute children, but only half the controls, were living with both parents. This was the case for 80% of the selectively mute children studied by Dummit et al. (1997). In individual case reports, when a couple have split up, the child's selective mutism has often predated the separation. For example, Tim (aged 5) was clearly not helped by his father leaving home unexpectedly a few months before his referral to a child guidance clinic, but his mother stressed that he had been refusing to speak at school for nearly a year before that (Sluckin,

1977). Some family case studies involve a family unit comprising mother, her new partner and the selectively mute child (e.g. Lindblad-Goldberg, 1986), but these are infrequent in the early clinical literature. Note, though, that some case studies have highlighted severe parental conflict (e.g. Woo, 1999) or multiple changes of carer (e.g. Tittnich, 1990) and that in one survey investigators have reported a higher incidence of parental separation and divorce (Black and Uhde, 1995). In a large survey by Ford et al. (1998) only 13% of respondents identified marital conflict as a key precipitating cause of selective mutism in their family. The authors concluded that their data failed 'to support notions that families of persons with SM have primarily negative characteristics' (p. 217).

The families of selectively mute children may generally stay together, but many of those described in the early clinical literature appear to have been quite unhappy. In some cases strong tensions and disharmony in parental relationships were reported. Communication between family members in clinic settings was often observed to be terse, constricted, and unsatisfying. Many early papers reflect the view of Subak, West and Carlin (1982) who described elective mutism in the title of their article as 'an expression of family psychopathology'. There must be some wariness in taking the often very negative accounts of family atmosphere in the literature at their face value. The main source is the observations of professionals working in clinic settings with rather little direct observation in the family home. When the parents are seen in their own home, shyness and lack of confidence often form a stronger impression on the interviewer than the tensions and emotional limitations described in some of the early literature.

The sparse survey evidence provides somewhat inconsistent evidence on the question of whether selectively mute children tend to live in households in which external social contacts are restricted. For example, Brown and Lloyd (1975) reported that, whereas only 49% of the families of the selectively mute children in their sample visited friends and relatives frequently, 83% of the families of control children did. The figures for visiting 'very rarely' or 'never' were 32% and 2% respectively. On the other hand, Ford et al. (1998) reported that the respondents to their survey most commonly described the families of selectively mute children as not just 'extremely close' but also 'socially active' (p. 215). It is difficult to interpret this finding, and further work is needed on the issue.

Key features of family structure in the analysis of some problems of social development are family size and birth order. In the case of selective mutism it is not clear whether these factors are relevant. The reports from different studies conflict. Brown and Lloyd (1975) found more selective mutism in large families and no significant relationships with birth order. Wright (1968) found just one only child in a series of 24 selectively mute children, yet Hesselman (1983) observed: 'In my other material . . . there are many families of only one or two children.' Kolvin and Fundudis

(1981) found no difference in family size between their selectively mute children and controls. They also found that selectively mute children tended to be born significantly early in their sibship. Wright (1968), on the other hand, highlighted the number of children in the middle of a sibship and suggested that in this context 'non-talking brought desired attention'. But Wilkins' (1985) data suggested that neither factor is relevant. In a survey of 100 cases Steinhausen and Juzi (1996) found rather a small number of only children and equal proportions of first-born and second- or later-born children. Neither birth order nor family size differentiated the selectively mute and control groups studies by Kristensen (2000). It seems likely that the development of selective mutism depends on subtle dynamic interactions that may occur equally in large or small families and at any point in a sibship (see later in the chapter – 'Sibling relationships').

Relationships between parents and children

In the early clinical literature the relationship of the parents of a selectively mute child was very occasionally described as warm and contented (e.g. Sluckin and Jehu, 1969). Generally, however, in clinic samples the parents' relationship was reported to be unhappy, tense and distrustful (Wright, 1968; Wilkins, 1985). Often one of the parents (usually the mother) was described as forming a coalition with the mute child in which the child 'serves as a shuttlecock of marital dissatisfaction' (Meyers, 1984) and the close relationship between mother and child is seen to be directly related to 'the hostile and disappointing relationship that the mother has with the father' (Browne, Wilson and Laybourne, 1963) or as a compensatory process that meets 'needs for closeness' that are not met by her husband (Tatem and DelCampo, 1995). Occasionally the marital problems were hidden, and the child's behaviour was seen as functioning to divert attention from them (e.g. Rosenberg and Lindblad, 1978).

'An abnormally strong and persistent bond of interdependence between the mother and child' was common in the series of cases reviewed by Kolvin and Fundudis (1981). This was also the most common pattern in Hayden's (1980) analysis of 68 loosely defined cases of selective mutism – a pattern she called 'symbiotic mutism'. The experience of interdependency between mother and child is vividly presented in the literature: both feel they cannot survive without the other (Meyers, 1984); the child repeatedly has difficulties in separating when starting Sunday School or nursery or school (Pustrom and Speers, 1964) or when the mother starts work (Wright et al., 1985, Case 1); the mother is seen as overprotective (Parker, Olsen and Throckmorton, 1960; Adams, 1970; Semenoff, Park and Smith, 1976; Meijer, 1979). When the child refuses to speak, the mother may be accepting and indulgent in her reaction (Sluckin and Jehu, 1969), whereas the father offers a more active response, such as attempting to bribe and bully the child to talk (Crema and Kerr, 1978). In a small number of cases the child refused to speak to any member of the family whom the mother rejected, such as the paternal grandfather (e.g. Meijer, 1979, Case 2) or, more commonly, the father (e.g. Ruzicka and Sackin, 1974).

Generally the closeness of mother and child was presented in the literature as pathological. In the light of recent work on behavioural inhibition the maternal stance may be re-interpreted as protective of a particularly vulnerable child. Sometimes it can be seen that a mother whose situation has placed her in this unusual relationship with her child has been enabled by it eventually to make insightful observations and effective moves to assist the child towards independence. For example, the team treating Mark (aged 9) at a residential centre discovered when his mother visited that she was already encouraging him to speak using non-verbal strategies that they had evolved over an extended period (Hill and Scull, 1985). Similarly, Mrs C invented a stimulus fading programme for her selectively mute daughter, Jenny, which was later adopted in a slightly more systematic form by a clinical team (Afnan and Carr, 1989). In any case it is always dangerous to generalize too confidently about maternal involvement and protectiveness. The straightforward picture of it that has been given above may be common, but there are exceptions in the case study literature. For example, Elson et al. (1965) described a series of four cases, all girls, in which the mother was rejecting of the children and the father detached and uninterested.

Fathers of selectively mute children have often been represented as detached from the issue. Sometimes this was because their work constantly took them away from the home, e.g. as a lorry driver or soldier. More often they were portrayed as simply not interested both by professionals (e.g. Elson et al., 1965) and by the young people themselves. A 13-year-old described by Wilkins (1985) said to his grandmother: 'Gran, would you care if I didn't talk to you? Dad doesn't care. No one cares.' The negative relationship between selectively mute children and their fathers is often just a matter of shyness and limited communication (e.g. Scott, 1977). Of the selectively mute children studied by Steinhausen and Juzi (1996), 11% did not speak to their fathers. Sometimes, however, the problems were more serious. Four of the 13 children reviewed by Koch and Goodlund (1973) expressed fear of their fathers at around the time of admission to hospital (cf. Charles in Adams and Glasner, 1954). It is not unusual in the literature for a negative spiral to be described in which the child's refusal to speak provokes an angry reaction from their father which inhibits further their readiness to speak with him (e.g. Crema and Kerr, 1978). The overt fear and timidity may conceal considerable anger. By the time Silverman and Powers (1970) saw Eric (aged 13) he was able to express this directly, though he had suppressed it in the past. His childhood in a family of eight children had been materially deprived, and he blamed his father who would abandon the household with great regularity.

The hurt may also be on the father's side. Meijer (1979) described a 9-year-old girl whose father 'had developed a paranoid system involving his wife and also his co-workers. He was a hypersensitive person who felt easily rejected and had isolated himself from all relatives. He blamed his wife for the child's symptom and for separating him from the children. He did not admit to violent physical attacks on his wife which she had mentioned, but accused her of maintaining family contacts which he had broken.' This account typifies the portrayal of the atmosphere within families of selectively mute children that was presented in the early clinical literature. The failure of recent clinical and research reports to examine family dynamics means that it is not possible to confirm the validity of such accounts as a general picture.

Sibling relationships

Rivalry and competition between siblings is a strikingly common feature in early accounts of selectively mute children (e.g. Koch and Goodlund, 1973; Wright et al., 1985). Very often there are exceptional difficulties in accepting the baby who is born when the child who later becomes mute is a toddler. For example, at the age of 16 months Amy, who was described by Chethik (1975), reacted to the birth of her brother Brad and her mother's subsequent period of depression by refusing to feed herself, fighting with her mother while resisting separation from her, physically attacking Brad who had to be protected, and refusing to sleep or to stay in her crib. Sometimes parents link the onset of mutism in time with the birth of the younger sibling (e.g. Adams, 1970; Afnan and Carr, 1989). A variant on this was reported by Youngerman (1979) who learned that his selectively mute patient, Owen, had given a hostile reaction initially to his younger sister's birth but did not express this through mutism until she started to speak when she was about 18 months and he was 3.

The incidence of selective mutism is heightened among the siblings of selectively mute children (e.g. Shaw, 1971; Baldwin, 1985). Emma, who was described by Wulbert et al. (1973), had four younger siblings who showed 'a similar pattern of selective responding'. In the Birmingham survey Brown and Lloyd (1975) found that there were twice as many children with a mute sibling in the selectively mute group as there were in the control group. In the sample of 30 children studied by Black and Uhde (1995) there were three selectively mute siblings from one family and two from another. Youngerman (1979) suggested that this may sometimes arise through imitation, but today workers in this field would be more likely to highlight genetic factors in this situation. At the same time siblings sometimes show contrasting problems, such as acting out (Ambrosino and Alessi, 1979) or shoplifting (Sluckin, 1977) or severe asthma (Meyers, 1984). The complex dynamics of relationships within a sibling group are well illustrated by the account given by Barlow, Strother and Landreth (1986) of sibling group therapy sessions aimed at helping

Amy, a selectively mute child aged 5. She came to most of the sessions with her two brothers, Ben who was 9 and Ned who was the youngest. In a key phase of the therapy (p. 48):

> Ben was gradually able to let Amy be her own person and retain his significant position of being one of several responsible members of the family. The mother encouraged this shift in communication at home by giving Amy more responsibility and not allowing Ben to take over her tasks, even when he could do them better and faster. Ned also maintained a balanced independence, rather than adopting Amy's role of being helpless and in total control or Ben's role of being responsible and in total control. Amy began to express feelings more frequently . . . (and her) new confidence extended into the classroom. Talking, singing and participating in class became fun for her.

Sibling interactions may sometimes play a direct role in the development of selective mutism. In two families known to SB the selectively mute child was a girl. In the first family the mother was German and the father was English. Both English and German were spoken at home. Rosa was the eldest of three and showed a high degree of shyness as a young child. She did not speak on entry to school, and this was not resolved through sessions of family therapy which took place over a year. She also refused to eat in school and waited until she was walking home from school before she would open her lunch box. A stimulus fading programme was carried out in different parts of the school. Initially she read to her mother alone, and then other children from her class joined them, at first singly and then in pairs. Rosa complied with this because of the variety of reinforcement she received, but showed her anger at a halfway point by encouraging her younger brother who was in his first term at school to keep silent there. Everyone was unsure why Peter had suddenly become mute, and there was great concern for the first 2 weeks of term until their mother noticed Rosa putting her finger to closed lips and signalling to him as they went into school. She dealt with this quickly and effectively, and continued to work with Rosa in school (A full account of stimulus fading can be found in Chapter 7).

In the second case, Lucy, an American child living in the UK, had not spoken in school since entry to nursery, although she spoke to one friend and to the child's mother at their home, in her home and in playgrounds where they were not overheard. A new assistant at the school was faded into the home setting. At the same time a parallel programme took place with Lucy, her mother and younger sister, Louisa, playing games in school after hours to encourage her to use her voice in the building. Although both children obtained small rewards for each step of Lucy's progress, Louisa seemed to resent the amount of attention Lucy was getting and stopped speaking at her nursery where she had previously been fairly talkative. The staff decided on a consistent policy of ignoring her when she did not speak. This resulted in a return to normal speaking after a difficult week of screaming and tantrums.

Although the pattern of sibling relationships was different, these cases underline the need to deal swiftly with the situation when a second child seems to develop patterns of non-speaking when the first child's difficulties are receiving attention.

Selective mutism in twins

> When I was small, I just didn't want to talk for some reason I don't know. Now I am older, I still don't know. I am afraid what people will say if I start now. (written by Joyce, aged 13)

> My reason is the same reason why my sister didn't talk. She didn't talk so I didn't talk. I don't know the reason. (written by her twin Ruth during the same clinic session and reported by Mora, De Vault and Schopler, 1962)

There have been other striking reports of the development of selective mutism in twins (e.g. Wallace, 1986). Although comparative incidence figures are not available, it is noticeable that twins appear fairly often in the literature. For example, two of the selectively mute children reviewed by Koch and Goodlund (1973) are said to have had competitive relationships with a twin, and there were three sets of twins altogether in their series of 13 selectively mute children. Two of three selectively mute children described by Halpern, Hammond and Cohen (1971) were twin girls, as were two of the six children described by Smayling (1959). It is an international phenomenon. For example, Tachibana et al. (1982) reported on Japanese twins who were selectively mute. At least 12 of the 302 children described in the published literature in English up to 1992 were twins, suggesting a minimum incidence of 4% (to be compared with the figure of 1:88 or 1.1% live births which represents the overall incidence of twins in the general child population – Schroeder, 1992).

The environment in which twins develop speech and language is different in significant respects from that of most children. Its most consistent pattern is a three-way exchange with an adult caretaker involving the other twin (Savic, 1980). The sharing of adults means that each twin receives less speech directed specifically to them than is the case for singleton children (Tomasello, Mannle and Kruger, 1986). They also spend more time speaking with their twin – another immature learner at an early stage of language development. The outcome is that, if the language of young twins is compared to the norms of singletons of the same age, they often appear to show a temporary delay (Lytton, Conway and Sauve, 1977). In addition, their speech often shows unique features shared by the two twins but not by others in their circle. One reason for this is that their language has to encompass concepts for which others have no equivalent and therefore no word – in particular, a concept of self-in-combination-with-twin as a psychological entity distinct from the individual self. For example, in a study of crib talk between identical girl twins Malmstrom and Silva (1986) observed a number of unusual features that appropriately expressed their twin status: they used a double name for themselves as a team ('Krista–Kelda' and 'Kelda–Krista'), while using the separate names, Kelda and Krista, to refer to themselves and each other individually; they used singular verbs in reference to themselves together; and they used the singular pronoun 'me' in reference to themselves as a team (e.g. 'Which one of me is this?' when showing a picture of one of the twins).

Typically, such usages are left behind as each twin develops a more confident separate individual identity. Waterman and Shatz (1982) argued that this aspect of their language development should not be described as delayed but rather as having some additional steps that are not found with other children. But for some twins the task of differentiating themselves from each other is too challenging to face. They may maintain a private language for an extended period (Thorpe et al., 2001), behave in ways that emphasize their closeness to the exclusion of others, and resist separation or even distinction between them. They may also, jointly, become selectively mute. For Joyce and Ruth whose mutism had been maintained for 8 years 'the symptom seemed to represent a kind of magic, symbolic tie between them which neither was able to break' (Mora, De Vault and Schopler, 1962). For June and Jennifer in their teens, talking to others would be a betrayal of each other (Wallace, 1986). For Denise and Diane (aged 6) 'the impetus for the mutism appears to have originated . . . within the twinship as part of a compact to maintain a fused identity' (Halpern, Hammond and Cohen, 1971).

These pairs of twins were not successful in suppressing their individual identities completely. Each pair had a member who sometimes gave adults signs of being almost ready to talk and a member who was dominant and had more invested in the exclusivity of the twinship. When an enforced trial separation was planned for June and Jennifer in the year before they left school, 'Jennifer knew this was her last chance to keep June for herself. 'You are Jennifer. You are me,' she would incant again and again. June's position was intolerable. She could not survive alone, but the price was to absorb Jennifer's identity. Tim Thomas (the educational psychologist) remembers her terrible cry: 'I am June. I am June,' as Jennifer forced her to submit.' (Wallace, 1986, p. 38) But neither twin found separation tolerable: it was June who had reacted most dangerously to the first attempt, refusing food, sitting in a rigid fixed pose for hours on end, weeping silently. It may appear that selective mutism in twins must be particularly resistant to treatment. No generalization is possible because of the very small number of cases on which published reports are available. But Halpern, Hammond and Cohen (1971) showed that with much younger children progress can be achieved fairly quickly. Issues of identity and competition within a twinship create an additional dimension. But, as in the case of language acquisition, the development of selective mutism in twins follows the same basic pattern as in other children.

The community

The family in the community

Selective mutism is not associated with any particular social class background (Wright, 1968). There may be a slight tendency for it to be more common in groups of lower socioeconomic status (Kopp and Gillberg, 1997; Andersson and Thomsen, 1998; Kristensen, 2000), but this may be because of other factors such as ethnicity or social isolation (Brown and Lloyd, 1975; Kolvin and Fundudis, 1981). Where researchers have reported a slight middle-class bias, this seems to have arisen from the use of a self-help group as a sample source (e.g. Steinhausen and Adamek, 1997). The families are sometimes described as being wary of the outside world. As noted above, survey evidence in the UK indicated that in one sample they went out together to visit friends or relatives markedly less often than the families of controls (Brown and Lloyd, 1975). A review of casework files in a US study suggested that the parents tended to be 'relatively inactive socially' (Parker, Olsen and Throckmorton, 1960). This is a feature noted in a number of individual case studies in the literature (e.g. Goll, 1979; Morin, Ladouceur and Cloutier, 1982; Kehle, Owen and Cressy, 1990), though not always confirmed in surveys (Ford et al., 1998).

In some cases isolation arises partly or mainly from living in a rural location that is remote from other households (e.g. Brison, 1966; Scott, 1977; Crema and Kerr, 1978; Baldwin, 1985). Often the key factor is not mainly geographical isolation but a social isolation that the family imposes on itself or on the child. Sally, who was described by Buck (1987), lived until she was 7 in an area of Canada where there were no close neighbours and the family was snowed in for five months of the year. Sally's parents managed to do their shopping by car, but socialized hardly at all. Sally's own social interactions were almost exclusively with her mother. The father in Family B described by Goll (1979) felt like an outsider in the small coastal town where they lived, because he maintained the traditional lifestyle of a sealhunter although the rest of the population had turned to more modern ways of making a living (cf. Morin, Ladouceur and Cloutier, 1982).

Sometimes it appears as though a child or parent prefers comparative isolation. For example, in early childhood 'K. always enjoyed playing alone on an open porch at the rear of the apartment in which her family lived. This allowed easy supervision by her mother, but deprived K. of the company and playtime with other children during her preschool years.' (Ambrosino and Alessi, 1979) A similar isolation was imposed on Norman, an only child, by his widowed mother (Morris, 1953). A whole household may reproduce such isolation even in an inner city environment. Lesser-Katz (1986) identified an unusually large number of selectively mute children in a Head Start preschool facility in a poor Chicago neighbourhood and related this in part to the tendency families showed 'to keep to themselves and to regard the environment outside their homes as hostile, or at least unfriendly'. As reported in Chapter 1, children from ethnic and linguistic minorities and from immigrant families show a relatively high incidence of selective mutism. This may be associated with situational factors that inhibit relaxed conversation, such as being the only black child in the class (Pigott and Gonzales, 1987) or speaking a language at home that is discouraged in school (Calhoun and Koenig, 1973). Sometimes one or more members of the family encourage the child to expect such problems. Goll (1979) employed the term 'ghetto family' to identify families with very little confidence in society, in which a selectively mute child experiences the boundary between their family and the outside world as a significant social barrier inhibiting free communication.

The child's relations with peers

When most children make their first regular independent ventures outside the home into the wider community, an important feature of the experience is forming new relationships with other children. This is a moment of crisis for some of those who become selectively mute. For example, they may show exceptional timidity or may react adversely to teasing. But many of the children form relaxed and apparently balanced relationships with a small number of friends. Communication with them may be odd, though. For example, Rebecca (aged 12) had never spoken a word at school. She had a number of friends from there with whom she often spent leisure time shopping or visiting one another's homes, but she did not speak to them in person, only on the telephone (Black and Uhde, 1992).

Nearly half the selectively mute children in the Finnish survey participated in activities with classmates in the classroom and during breaks (Kumpulainen et al., 1998). Some selectively mute children surprise adults by being quite assertive with their peers (Wright et al., 1985). It has often been reported that even those who do form friendships show immature social skills within them. A 5-year-old seen by Meijer (1979) was often provocative towards peers in the nursery and would sometimes yell derogatory remarks at them. John, aged 12, would stand on the edge of a group, unable to make the appropriate moves to join in their games although obviously wishing to do so (Wassing, 1973).

Peers often appear to collude with and reinforce a child's mute behaviour in a number of ways – by acknowledging its interest value, showing genuine concern, giving the child protection and support, taking collective responsibility for the child's lack of speech by interpreting the child's needs to adults such as teachers (Edmondson, 1986). Sometimes most pupils ignore a selectively mute child but one or two motherly girls function as supporters and interpreters. Cora (aged 7) was physically rigid as well as mute in school. 'At recess time there was a whole ritual attached to Cora's leaving the classroom. Someone would first touch her to indicate that it was time to leave. Another child would shove her into her sweater. Another would touch her back to indicate that she was to go out-side' (Landgarten, 1975). A selectively mute child's interpreter may gain special status and some power from the role and may resist giving it up. Winter (1984) and others have turned this round in school-based behav-iour management by appointing 'peer therapists' with a special responsibility to reinforce speech. This is discussed in more detail in Chapter 4.

It will be evident that the quality of the research base for different sec-tions of this chapter has been quite uneven. There have been great advances in recent years in what is understood about characteristics of the individual child with selective mutism, but there has been much less work on the systems of family and community in which the child is placed and which may be assumed to have an influence on how a problem of com-munication develops. In the next chapter we examine models of the development of selective mutism. For that purpose it is necessary to con-sider both the children and their situation in a family and a community.

Chapter 3
The development of selective mutism

Selective mutism may develop in many different ways. This chapter presents an analysis of the factors that dispose a child to be vulnerable, the factors that precipitate mutism in some settings, and the factors that then serve to maintain this pattern of behaviour once it is established. Earlier clinical investigators working within the therapeutic framework of a psychodynamic or behavioural or family therapy perspective focused on intrapsychic and family dynamics and on individual patterns of behaviour. With this orientation they often ignored two issues that have emerged as crucial in recent research:

- the genetic predisposition of a child who becomes selectively mute
- ways in which the family and the child transact their relationships with external systems.

A full account of the development of selective mutism must encompass all the systems that are involved in the child's life.

In the past it was generally accepted that the aetiology of selective mutism was heterogeneous. For example, Halpern, Hammond and Cohen (1971) and Meijer (1979) each set out long lists of causative factors identified in the literature. This lack of consensus led some commentators to cast doubt on the status of the term. Youngerman (1979) argued that elective mutism denotes 'neither a diagnostic term nor a defined syndrome but simply a descriptive label (that) . . . collects a disparate patient population under a single rubric'. During the 1980s and early 1990s the focus on behavioural approaches led many investigators to ignore historic aetiology in their concern to attend to maintaining factors in the child's current situation. But, although an argument could be made for this as a legitimate strategy for planning intervention in a specific case, a full general account of the phenomenon cannot be given without attention to how it develops.

During the last decade there has been increasing interest in the possibility that children who develop selective mutism start with a predisposition or vulnerability to problems of that kind. This line of thinking was given an impetus by the recent work on behavioural inhibition and temperamental shyness that was described in the previous chapter. Predisposing factors for selective mutism are the subject of a central section in this chapter. But it seems unlikely that these factors operate alone in most cases of selective mutism. Although there may be indications of a shy and inhibited temperament from very early in infancy, it is likely that external factors play a part in precipitating and maintaining the use of silence in selected situations (Dow et al., 1995).

One factor will be that, since the children's temperamental tendencies have familial roots, there will almost certainly be some transmission of anxiety between parents and children, affecting their approach to the unfamiliar. More direct consequences of having an anxious temperament are likely to include that at an early stage certain common childhood challenges such as separation anxiety, fear of the unfamiliar, embarrassment and fear of failing are experienced in acute forms. For example, as we noted in Chapter 1, parents of children who are selectively mute are often reported to have said that an adverse early separation experience had left a scar on them and their child amounting to a 'trauma'.

Some authors have characterized different subtypes of selective mutism, referring to differences in aetiology as well as presenting behaviour. The example of Reed (1963) was discussed above. Another example was Hayden (1980) whose work has been treated cautiously because she employed an over-inclusive definition of the phenomenon. However, her analysis of subtypes remains of interest in illustrating the potential benefits and risks of this kind of approach to analysing the condition. She described four subtypes:

- **symbiotic mutism:** characterized by a symbiotic relationship with a caretaker and by a submissive but manipulative relationship with others
- **speech phobic mutism:** characterized by fear of hearing one's own voice and by use of ritualistic behaviours
- **reactive mutism:** characterized by withdrawal and depression which apparently resulted from trauma
- **passive-aggressive mutism:** characterized by hostile use of silence as a weapon.

Hayden's analysis shows the advantages of highlighting the association between particular patterns of aetiology and particular patterns of behaviour. However, in selective mutism the patterns are not as clearcut as she suggested. For example, the rich and complex portrait she herself gives of Kevin in *Murphy's Boy* (Hayden, 1983) belies the possibility of fitting individuals neatly into the diagnostic sub-categories she had presented in her earlier paper. At one moment or another many selectively mute children present one or other of the behaviour patterns which she describes, moving between them. There is no evidence for interpreting them separately as 'types'.

Whatever the aetiology behind the initial onset of mutism, new factors may operate to maintain and develop it once the pattern is established. Some of the accounts of young people in their teens who have been selectively mute for a number of years present a picture of complex and deep-seated emotional disturbance with a wide range of deviant behaviour patterns. For example, Owen (aged 14) who had been selectively mute since the age of 3 had recently become mute even at home, refused to wash, and would not part with old torn clothing. He would lock himself in the family's only bathroom for 45 minutes at a time (Youngerman, 1979). Sara (also aged 14) refused not only to talk but also to walk. She arrived at the residential centre with her mother's left arm crooked around her shoulders. At each step her mother would push one of her knees in turn from behind with her free hand. 'Sara moved slowly, allowing her mother to push each leg about two inches forward with each touch of the knee.' (Roberts, 1984) Thus elaborate rituals and extreme forms of manipulation of members of the family develop on the back of the determined refusal to talk that has lasted for many years (often with short breaks after partially successful treatment). The young person's social isolation and inability to respond adaptively to the new challenges of early adolescence create an impetus for the pattern of mutism to broaden to other areas of personal and social functioning. This section will mainly deal with the aetiology of early onset selective mutism. But those working with older clients have to take account of the overlay of later features. Other reports of selective mutism and its sequelae in adolescence include Kaplan and Escoll (1973), Munford et al. (1976), Kupietz and Schwartz (1982), Eldar et al. (1985), Wilkins (1985), Tibbles and Russell (1992).

Predisposing factors

There is evidence from one survey (as yet not confirmed by others) that children who later become selectively mute share a pattern of risk factors with other child psychiatric patients. For example, they are more likely than the majority of children to have encountered complications during pregnancy, delivery and the neonatal period (Steinhausen and Juzi, 1996). However, the most significant findings in this field do not concern non-specific risk factors but patterns of genetic predisposition that relate more closely to the pattern of deviant behaviour that develops later (Steinhausen and Adamek, 1997). In the previous chapter we outlined recent thinking on the temperamental characteristic of behavioural inhibition to which an increasingly important role in the development of selective mutism has been attributed over the last decade.

The initial reason for that attribution can be readily appreciated if one reads an account of how many children behave at the age of 3 after their mothers leave them on their first day at nursery school:

All showed behaviour defined as automanipulation (fingering or rubbing mouth, nose, ears or hair, or some small object which they did not look at). All but one showed periods of immobility accompanied by fixed gaze . . . About one third chewed or mouthed objects or fingers and one child rocked. In response to eye contact the new child glanced or looked away (usually down) . . . sidling locomotion and shuffling were common while standing still.

(McGrew, 1972)

This is a good description of the observed behaviour of young selectively mute children faced with uncertainty and unfamiliarity.

Inhibition of motor activity is a biologically determined initial response to uncertainty. In 2–3 year olds, as illustrated in that account, this may be shown in stopping play, becoming quiet and seeking a familiar source of comfort (or showing distress if none is available). Kagan, Reznick and Snidman (1987) suggested that this is a sensitive time to identify behavioural tendencies towards inhibition or lack of inhibition to the unfamiliar. These results have been replicated in other studies with children ranging from infants to 11-year-olds. The children who show extremely inhibited or uninhibited behaviour early are more likely to retain this pattern in later childhood. There is disagreement on the question of whether inhibition should be thought of dimensionally (i.e. as though inhibited children are on a continuum) (Kerr et al., 1994) or categorically (i.e. as though inhibited and uninhibited children are qualitatively distinct) (Kagan, Reznick and Snidman, 1987). For those concerned with selective mutism that is a less crucial issue than the question of whether behavioural inhibition in infancy is a necessary precursor of the development of selective speech refusal. Not all inhibited children develop selective mutism, but parents' retrospective accounts of the infancy of selectively mute children often describe a quiet, cautious, easily startled personality. It is also clear that not all children who have been selectively mute develop anxiety disorders, but as adults they may still see themselves as rather shy and reserved.

It has been argued that the temperamental construct of behavioural inhibition could be linked with the behavioural inhibition system (BIS) in Gray's neuropsychological model (1987, 1988). Much of his theorizing was based on animal studies in which anxiolytic drugs were shown to have the effect of diminishing activity in the BIS. Overactivity in the brain was associated with pathological anxiety. The BIS responds to three kinds of stimuli: (1) novel stimuli, (2) signals of impending punishment, and (3) stimuli which signal non-reward, i.e. the omission of anticipated reward or the termination of reward. The last two are seen as threatening or aversive. Activity in the BIS may produce various changes: inhibition of all ongoing behaviour, increased attention to the environment, especially any new features, and a raised level of arousal. In Gray's model, an opposing system, the behavioural activating system (BAS), is sensitive to signals of reward and stimuli that signal the ending or omission of punishment. Activity in the BAS is thought to give rise to positive emotional states and, at a high level of activity, to impulsive behaviour.

There is some evidence from studies employing various 'stop' tasks that children with anxiety disorders who show a strong inhibitory response have high levels of BIS activity (Oosterlaan, 2001). An overfunctioning BIS may be a pathway by which temperamental inhibition leads to the development of anxiety disorders, though there may be other pathways too (Turner, Beidel and Wolff, 1996). However, an extreme level of activity in the BIS which increases sensitivity to novelty, as well as to cues that signal punishment or non-reward, could specifically produce conditioning that would generate avoidance and the development of anxious behaviour. Inhibition may be one factor which predisposes the development of anxiety, or, on the hypothesis that an overfunctioning BIS plays a part, it may just represent an enhanced risk. Although the development of anxiety disorders will ultimately depend on other environmental and cognitive influences, the children's genetic inheritance of a highly active BIS may be a significant risk factor. Identifying children who show extreme and persistent temperamental inhibition may give opportunities for effective early intervention.

A different line of investigation has been suggested by Hagerman et al. (1999) who described a case study of a 12-year-old girl with fragile X syndrome who had a long history of social anxiety, shyness and selective mutism. Fragile X syndrome is a genetic syndrome caused by a defect on the X chromosome. Children with fragile X often appear normal in infancy but later develop typical physical characteristics such as prominent ears. They often have moderate or severe learning difficulties. Hagerman et al. argued that, as shyness and social anxiety are often associated with this syndrome, it may be an undiagnosed feature of selective mutism in many cases. They recommended that children with selective mutism should be tested for it 'particularly if they have language and/or cognitive deficits or a family history of SM, autism or mental retardation' (p. 316).

Simons, Goode and Fombonne (1997) highlighted a different abnormality when they reported on a 4-year-old girl who was selectively mute at nursery. Chromosome analysis indicated that there was a deletion of the short arm of chromosome 18. Her parents did not show the same abnormality, and it was difficult to interpret the significance of this isolated finding. No other research teams have replicated these case study findings, and for the present there is an overwhelming argument for focusing on behavioural inhibition as a possible factor.

These are predisposing factors within the child. There may also be predisposing factors at the level of the family and the community. These are discussed below in the section on ecological perspectives on selective mutism.

Events that precipitate the onset of mutism

For most of the children who are described as selectively mute, a key moment is said to have been when they started at nursery or school. For some the school situation stimulates anxiety that causes a strong adverse reaction. For others the school situation merely offers a new stage on which an already established pattern of behaviour is shown up as inescapably unusual and problematic. For both groups the school setting adds considerably to earlier challenges that the child has faced. It requires regular separation from the mother, and it imposes continuous demands to speak that are outside the child's control. Of course, as Brown and Lloyd (1975) showed, many children do not talk easily when they start school, but most overcome this. An adequate theory of the aetiology of selective mutism must explain how that process is inhibited in a small number of children.

The precipitating factor is not always starting at school. Sometimes the onset of mute behaviour dates from another separation from mother – she starts regular work (Wright et al., 1985) or goes into hospital (Adams, 1970). A key factor may be the acceptability of the arrangements for substitute care. The boy described by Adams was sent for 10 days to stay with a hostile grandmother who farmed him out with a neighbour. The list of traumatic experiences associated with the onset of mutism goes beyond straightforward separations. Almost one in five of respondents to one survey recalled that they had moved home during the year prior to starting school (Ford et al., 1998). Or the source of upset may be more personal: Tessa (aged 4) was forced to see a doctor after being promised that that would not happen (Sluckin and Jehu, 1969). In one case the supposed precipitating event was being instructed to be quiet at the house of the mother's employer (Koch and Goodlund, 1973). These authors suggested that where there is a precipitating event of this kind there may be a higher chance of a positive outcome.

An emphasis on a single precipitating event is encouraged by the truism that for everyone there is probably 'a threshold of how much tension and anxiety the child can tolerate and still be able to speak' (Gemelli, 1983). Some parents find comfort in identifying a particular supposedly traumatic event as the cause of the child's behaviour. In some accounts what is then described is a reaction that does not amount to selective mutism as defined in Chapter 1. One of the children reviewed by Parker, Olsen and Throckmorton (1960) was mute for a short time after his father had died and his mother had moved the family from an isolated farm to a medium-sized town. Another two followed a similar pattern after they had been separated from their mothers when they (the mothers) were hospitalized (cf. Gemelli, 1983, p. 20.)

For some children whose selective mutism has lasted for much longer there seems little doubt that a crucial precipitating factor has been a traumatic event in or around the family – for K (aged 5) her father's stroke and death (Ambrosino and Alessi, 1979), for Jean (aged 6) the death of the grandmother with whom she had been living for most of her early life (Sluckin, 1977) (cf. Mora, De Vault and Schopler, 1962). In general, however, there is no such dramatic change or loss in the lives of children who become selectively mute. Typically the onset of the behaviour is slow and insidious. It comes to the fore when they face new social challenges that exacerbate or highlight what is already evident to those closest to them, most often the challenge of starting school or nursery.

Accounts in the psychodynamic and behavioural traditions

Most discussion of aetiology until the last two decades was within one of the two main theoretical traditions – psychodynamic and behavioural. That history may be traced clearly in the literature reviews by Kratochwill (1981) and Hesselman (1983). Both traditions accept some core features in the development of selective mutism as far as the children themselves are concerned:

- They show a lack of age-appropriate independence from their families or, more particularly, from their mothers. In social learning they tend to rely on models within the family.
- Their relationships to family members often have an oppositional quality and reveal a vein of obstinacy.
- There is a sense of threat outside the family, or at least of some difficulties in dealing with the outside world. The perception of this by the child is an important factor in the initial refusal to speak.
- Secondary gains play a part in determining children's persistence in maintaining their silence.

Beyond this limited common ground the theorists in the two traditions have predictably chosen a quite different focus of attention. Those within the psychodynamic tradition have usually explained the children's selective silence by a detailed analysis of the course of their psychosexual development. In a typical formulation the mutism has been seen as 'a protective mechanism . . . a fixation at an early infantile level, on which an apprehended danger situation is met by a refusal to speak' (Salfield, 1950). Because of their mother's personal depression or rejection of them, the children are unable to acknowledge hostile feelings towards her or to express those feelings directly. They remain dependent on her and unable to make normal moves towards independence. They fear separation and abandonment. Their hostility is safely expressed through passively hostile behaviour towards third parties such as teachers or other adults rather than towards the true object, the mother. The primary gain is that the children are relieved of the anxiety associated with the unexpressed hostility and rage. The secondary gains are that they can enjoy continued dependency and received increased attention because of their behaviour (Elson et al., 1965).

There are important differences of view within the tradition. Writers have differed in when they believe the arrest of development occurs, some emphasizing the anal stage rather than the oral stage. Others have rejected the notion that there will be a consistent link between the genesis of selective mutism and a particular stage of psychosexual development. They have emphasized instead the meanings silence accumulates for a child over time and suggested that the behaviour 'often synthesizes conflicts from many different developmental levels' (Chethik, 1975). Why is the child's conflict expressed through not talking? To explain this it is necessary to return to first principles and recall the role of language in child development. 'Words label first the outer and then the inner world, permitting that crucial distinction between reality and fantasy' which is basic to the development of thinking processes (Youngerman, 1979). He goes on to quote from the manifesto of a selectively mute young person from Belgium:

- One doesn't speak because one doesn't want to bind oneself to others by the word . . .
- One doesn't speak because whoever gives us a chance to pull out of our isolation is an intruder.
- One doesn't speak because in the end, in life, one is alone, even if one speaks.
- One does not speak because one has not had Mama's smile.

Formulations within the behavioural tradition stress the consequences of the behaviour that might be experienced as positive by the child – fear and anxiety reduced, unpleasantness avoided, and privileges and attention gained (Hesselman, 1983). The mutism may be seen as negatively reinforced through the avoidance of speech demands that make the child anxious (e.g. Sluckin, 1977). Processes of social modelling may be highlighted: the child adopts attitudes and behaviours that are prevalent within the family (e.g. Scott, 1977). Many authors in this tradition have emphasized the importance of factors that maintain the child's mutism once it is established. The mutism will be reinforced if adults accept and facilitate the lack of verbal responses (e.g. Nolan and Pence, 1970) and if peers speak for the mute individual (e.g. Straughan, Potter and Hamilton, 1965). Attention has also been paid to how children interpret the reactions of others to their mutism and to the 'feedback' functions of the rewards children receive for speaking and for staying silent (e.g. Lachenmeyer and Gibbs, 1985).

Ecological perspectives

There is a serious problem about almost all the formulations described so far: they ignore the fact that selective mutism normally occurs outside the family. Developmental theories in psychology require an ecological dimension. An adequate theory will not just explain why a particular child develops a particular pattern of behaviour after particular early experiences. The theory will also explain why that pattern is found in particular situations. In the case of selective mutism what is required is a model that considers not only the child and the family but also their negotiated relationships with the outside world. This perspective has been reflected in the literature from an early stage. For example, Adams and Glasner (1954) described the behaviour as 'a defence mechanism . . . a means of avoiding a difficult environment . . . a barrier to protect themselves from the intrusion of a hostile, threatening world'. In the words of Goll (1980), it is as though the children 'have been inoculated with the idea that the outer world and its inhabitants are formidable and alarming'. Mutism is a strategy by which the child can guard against these dangerous forces, or control them (Pustrom and Speers, 1964). But what determines which particular situations will be treated by a child in this way?

Meyers (1984) presented a family systems approach to understanding selective mutism. She highlighted the involvement of the family in the complex aetiology of the child's behaviour and suggested that it was based in 'parent mutist modelling, family cultural tradition, symbiotic attachment, separation anxiety and poor marital adjustment. The family comprises a tightly knit social system where significant emotional exchanges are self-contained and where there is a generalized fear of strangers and the outside world.' Lindblad-Goldberg (1986) took these notions a step further, employing a model developed by Minuchin and his associates to describe psychosomatic illness in childhood (Table 3.1).

This open systems model is intended to emphasize the feedback systems between children who are selectively mute and their context. Lindblad-Goldberg's key assumptions are 'that (i) the family's organization and relationship to its extrafamilial context is closely related to the development and maintenance of elective mutism in children, and (ii) the elective mute's refusal to speak plays a major role in maintaining family homeostasis'. It is proposed that the child's mute behaviour plays a role in helping the family to avoid having to face up to or resolve internal conflicts. This means that the mute behaviour is constantly reinforced by the actions of other family members as well as by the child's own anxieties and secondary gains. A unique element in this family systems model is the proposal that 'the family experiences a developmental crisis whenever it reaches a point in the family life cycle that requires an increased exchange between the family and the extrafamilial environment'. Rooted in a family therapy tradition, this model explicates the family context of selective mutism confidently, and it offers a clearer account of systemic factors

Table 3.1 Parents' behaviour and the development of mutism

Parents' behaviour that is seen as supporting the development of selective mutism	References
Fail to expect or demand speech when the child is young	Adams and Glasner (1954)
Model silence as a reaction to strangers	Pustrom and Speers (1964) (Case 2) Sluckin (1977)
Put intense emotion into warnings against talking to strangers	Pustrom and Speers (1964) (Case 1) Sluckin and Jehu (1969)
Show a ready understanding of the child's mutism virtually amounting to collusion	Meijer (1979) (Case 4)
Fail to see the behaviour pattern as a problem	Albert-Stewart (1986) Winter (1984)
Yield very readily to the child's preferences rather than provoke a tantrum	Halpern et al. (1971) (Case 1)
Fail to develop a social life outside the family or model simple social transactions for the child	Brown and Lloyd (1975)
Use silence to express anger within the family	Meyers (1984)

within families than any earlier attempt. However, it does not offer much help in locating the child's and the family's behaviour in a wider social context, which we feel is of crucial importance.

In a more recent formulation Stein et al. (2001) attempted to highlight the importance of what he termed 'environmental change' in precipitating selective mutism. Stein's conceptualization of a pathway leading to selective mutism is shown in Table 3.2. This figure goes some way to acknowledging the significance of factors outside the family, but does not fully take into account the broader social and communal context of child development.

A further limitation of Stein's figure is that it does not take account of the impact of parents' own social anxiety and their previous experiences on how they deal with situations they face in their children's schools and how they are seen there. A negative cycle can develop in which parents who experience difficulty when meeting new people are seen as 'uncommunicative' by teachers. Then their anxiety increases because they are aware of how they are viewed . . . and so on. Anxiety may also cause the misinterpretation of social cues. Thus for some families school may become an 'extrafamilial environment' which is particularly difficult to deal with.

Table 3.2 Conceptualized pathway to selective mutism

Temperament	+	Family history of anxiety behaviours	+	Environmental change	➤	Selective mutism
shyness		excessive worries		new school		
worry		separation problems		new sibling		
social avoidance		tachycardia		marriage discord		
fearfulness		palpitations		family move		
social withdrawal		phobias		family illness		
clinging		hypervigilance				
negativism		social avoidance				

Source: Stein et al. (2001).

In addition, for some immigrant parents the schools that their children attend may have a very different ethos from the schools they attended themselves. There may be additional sources of challenge around language and curriculum differences.

Goll (1980) offered an influential formulation of how communal as well as intrafamilial factors may play a part in the aetiology of selective mutism. He argued that two main factors are required if selective mutism is to develop – a society that is able to produce and maintain outsiders and outsider groups, and a ghetto family that has very little confidence in society. He proposed that the family of a selectively mute child might include individuals playing four special roles:

- the selectively mute child
- a mutist model (or models) from whom the child learns to use stubborn silence as a strong weapon
- a symbiotic partner with whom the child enjoys or suffers an intense mutual dependency
- a ghetto leader who represents this marginalized family to the outside world which they perceive as not to be trusted.

This depiction of specific roles within the family has not been empirically validated on other samples, and 'role-spotting' may not be useful in trying to help an individual family. However, the model may be useful heuristically in suggesting both how the children in general may come to have a problem about communication and how the refusal to talk comes to be focused on settings in the wider community beyond the family. Goll's account also suggests some of the reasons why selective mutism may occur more often among ethnic minority and immigrant communities.

Analogous factors may operate in quite different settings. For example, Looff (1971) provides a vivid example of the fertile conditions for selective mutism in isolated rural communities in the Southern Appalachians in eastern Kentucky. There is a cultural tradition of taciturnity (of being 'quiet-turned'), and there is also a great social distance between the homes of many children and the schools in local towns and larger villages. That in itself would not be sufficient to foster selective mutism. But a few of the children who were exceptionally close to their mothers, and were discouraged by them from speaking to strangers, responded with persist-ent silent withdrawal. Looff's account is discussed in more detail in Chapter 4. As we shall see, the particular challenges that Goll and Looff described are likely to be experienced by many families and not just by those from minority ethnic backgrounds and isolated rural areas.

Table 3.3 presents a summary of how selective mutism may develop, making clear that the community as well as the child and the family may play a part in the process. It also differentiates between disposing factors that create a situation that is favourable to this development, precipitating factors that trigger the behaviour on the first few occasions, and main-taining factors that encourage its persistence. Selective mutism appears to be most likely when some factors are present at each of the levels (the community, the family and the child), but it may occur when only two lev-els are implicated. Tables 3.4, 3.5 and 3.6 set out specific examples of disposing, precipitating and maintaining factors, showing how related features may occur at each level. The planning of intervention discussed in Chapters 7 and 8 needs to take account of the range of factors at dif-ferent levels shown in these tables.

Table 3.3 A summary of how selective mutism may develop

	Community	Family	Child
Disposing factors	Family is isolated or marginalized in the community	Parents have personal experience and/or a family tradition of silence/reticence	Child has the temperamental charac-teristics of behavioural inhibition
		Factors within the family encourage mutism as a reac-tion to challenge	Factors within the child favour mutism as a reaction to challenge
Precipitating factors			The child faces a challenging transition to the outside world (or other stressful challenge) and reacts by withholding speech
Maintaining factors	Reactions from adults and peers reinforce mutism	Reactions from family members reinforce mutism	The child experiences reduced anxiety and secondary gains

Table 3.4 Possible disposing factors, which may also later serve a maintaining function

Community	Family	Child
Social distance maintained between families or groups in a rural community or between ethnic or linguistic groups in an urban community	A family history of shyness or mutism or social isolation	A temperamental disposition towards shyness, timidity and fearfulness ('behavioural inhibition')
	Modelling/encouragement of shyness or mutism by family members individually or as a whole group	Learning from family models
Community pressures, such as racial harassment (or simply a failure to welcome newcomers), foster family's sense of threat and isolation	Family ethos of group exclusivity and wariness in dealing with the outside world	
	Anxiety about disclosure of family secrets	
	Family unable to face and resolve conflicts	A strong need to control
		Negativism
	Marital problems and a strong bond of interdependence between mother and child, excluding or distancing father	Failure to develop age-appropriate independence from one or both parents
Peers who tease and reject those who are different (e.g. in speech mannerisms and/or accent)	Intense sibling rivalry	Speech difficulties

Table 3.5 Possible precipitating factors

Community	Family	Child
	Birth of a resented younger sibling (or their development of speech)	
	Family members cannot work through change or loss by sharing their feelings or open discussion	Is thrust into a new domestic situation without adequate preparation (e.g. after bereavement)
Legal requirement that all children attend school	Some family members find it extremely difficult when it is necessary for them or other family members to move outside the family circle	Starts nursery, play-group or school
	Family moves to new (and strange) environment, e.g. as immigrants	

Table 3.6 Possible maintaining factors

Community	Family	Child
Treat the child as special and unusual	Treat the child as special and unusual	Relishes own uniqueness Gains privileges and attention
Convey expectation that the child will remain mute	Convey expectation that the child will remain mute	Holds a self-image as a mute
		Is fearful of conse-quences of speaking
Reinforce non-verbal methods of communica-tion and make them effective, even in school	Reinforce non-verbal methods of communication and make them effective	Finds that silence need not bring social isolation or academic failure
	Experience reduced anxiety as the child's behaviour helps the family avoid having to resolve internal conflicts	Anxiety is reduced

Chapter 4
Education

In contrast to the numerous descriptions of selectively mute children and their families, very little has been written about the school context in which the behaviour occurs or on its effect on teachers and others in school. This chapter sets the context by outlining the school's role in socialization and teachers' expectations of children on school entry. It then examines processes in schools which reinforce and maintain mutism. The presence of a mute child has a powerful effect on teachers' feelings and often generates intense reactions. In this situation the teachers need emotional and practical support that is often not available. Yet many of the most successful methods of helping selectively mute children are school based.

The age of most selectively mute children at referral for help is closely related to the time of starting school. There are no published data on the incidence of selective mutism in nurseries and playgroups. Relatively few referrals are recorded in the literature, but they are not unknown (e.g. Tittnich, 1990). In addition, investigators frequently report retrospective comments about a child not having spoken in nursery. An increasing number of children are now entering their first educational setting at around their third birthday, a stage when many are not confident speakers, especially to people outside the home. Discussion with nursery teachers suggests that a number of children speak very little in nursery and that it is not uncommon for them to take a term to start talking in a relaxed way with adults.

Expectations shift as children approach school age. Some leeway is allowed to a preschool child. Parents will apologize for a young child who fails to respond to an approach from another adult: 'He's not himself today'. Popular idiom has other similar let-out phrases, such as 'Has the cat got your tongue, then?'. This is not only a defence of the child but a face saver for the adult who has been rebuffed.

The family's view of school and preparation of children for starting school is especially important if other aspects of the children's behaviour have caused concern. For example, 'You won't be able to do that when you go to school' or 'You'll have to talk properly when you go to school'. Starting school takes some children away from the only group of people with whom they have had practice in talking. For some the challenge of separation from their mother and the familiar setting of the home is over-whelming. The effect on some children is observable immediately.

The school's role in socialization

The significance of school entry age as the peak time for referral has been mentioned already. This is associated with the school's role in the social-ization of young children. In the past, when all the entrants began school together, starting school was often a distressing experience for many chil-dren. Teachers of reception classes used to spend the first weeks settling crying children and reassuring anxious mothers. Nowadays new children visit their school at least once before starting, and admissions may be spaced over several weeks so that the teacher has time to concentrate attention on each new arrival. Parents are welcomed into the school, and efforts are made to make them, as well as the children, feel 'at home' and part of the school community. As a result of all these measures, it is rare to find a child who shows open and prolonged distress over starting school (Cleave et al., 1982; Grannell, Hinton and O'Kelly, 1991).

Alongside this more gentle approach to welcoming parents and chil-dren into school, teachers still assume that the children will be 'ready for school'. The information booklets given to parents emphasize independ-ent self-care skills, dressing, mealtime behaviour and toilet habits as important ways in which parents can help their children to prepare for school. Approaches which encourage parents and children to give a pen picture of the children and their likes and dislikes assume a degree of lan-guage skill and social confidence. It is usually assumed that children will have had some preschool experience outside the home, will have experi-enced some separation from their mothers and will be accustomed to the company of other children.

It is not always easy for parents to give teachers information about their children which they feel is important. The entry forms that parents are asked to fill in before their children start show great variation between nurseries. Some forms ask for the minimum information – name, address, telephone number, place of work plus some health-related questions. Others encourage parents to give a pen picture of the children's favourite activities and ask about any special needs, often with reference to lan-guage skills. A smaller number go further and ask more open-ended questions covering children's feelings as well as their skills and interests. 'How confident is he about being understood when he talks?' ' Is there anything that particularly worries or frightens her?' 'How do you comfort him if he's upset?' Some establishments include in the form separate sheets for children themselves, e.g. a sheet with pictures of toys and activities in the nursery so that the children can colour the ones they like. Parents who experience this two-way process generally value it: 'I felt that they really wanted me to tell them about him because I know him best.'

Describing the process of socialization Kanner (1947) wrote of 'the branching out of the children's contacts in the community at about 4 to 5 years of age . . . The child's horizon expands with the meeting of other children and adults outside the family group.' The growth of playgroup and nursery provision may have brought this stage forward for many families. Whenever it occurs, a crucial factor in the process is children's ability to make their wants known and to reply to questions: the command of language and confidence in its use are the basis of social independence.

In the past it was not uncommon for children in remote rural areas to experience many problems on school entry. Looff (1971) provided a vivid example of such an area in his account of the Manchester project in eastern Kentucky. Children with emotional and behavioural problems could be referred to the project's 'field clinics' for help. Analysing project records he found a higher number of electively mute children than expected (2.8% of the case load of the field clinics), and he suspected that there were many more who had not been referred. If his statistics were compared with others in the US literature, he concluded, elective mutism in children 'would have a higher prevalence in the Southern Appalachian region than anywhere else in the nation.' He argued that one factor contributing to this phenomenon was a generally low level of verbal communication among many families in the area. There were both silent individuals, known locally as 'quiet-turned', and silent families where active practical skills were valued more than talk. This was especially true of the men, and Looff points out that boys would be trained from an early age to keep quiet on hunting and fishing expeditions.

Obviously this strong local cultural tradition had a significant influence in generating the conditions for Looff's findings of a high rate of referral of selectively mute children. But he identified a second important factor relating to school organization. An acute problem arose for some children when tiny schools with one, two or three rooms in isolated communities were closed and new 'consolidated elementary schools' opened to cater for more than 300 pupils in a whole district. Many children were unused to travelling outside their immediate community. For some the experience was overwhelming. 'In the classroom they remained frozen in their seats, would not say a word, and refused to move to go to the bathroom, lunchroom or playground. A few sobbed quietly as they sat. Several furtively nibbled at lunches brought from home, ceasing when noticed. None attempted to read or write.' According to previous school reports all these children had been considered extreme social isolates by their neighbours, but had been able to function in their former schools. The children's withdrawal, which persisted for 2–3 months, seemed to be an attempt to cope with the overwhelming anxiety of the unfamiliar situation. Similar accounts of selective mutism in children from rural areas may be found in Morris (1953) and Goll (1980).

Today in developed countries the isolation of such families is likely to be because of psychological, cultural and language factors rather than physical or geographical ones. The raised incidence of selective mutism in children from ethnic and linguistic minorities has already been mentioned. Selectively mute children have been reported more frequently in the recent past in towns and cities, particularly in districts where isolated mothers feel the need to impose a similar isolation on their children for the sake of safety. It may be relevant that many of the transactions of everyday life, such as shopping and paying the rent, are now commonly completed in relatively impersonal settings – a shift that is epitomized in the replacement of corner shops by large supermarkets. In atomized urban communities, as in scattered rural communities, the school faces particular challenges in its role as a focus for communal socialization.

Preventive work with behaviourally inhibited children

A significant proportion of children will feel shy and intimidated when they start at playgroup, nursery or school, and within this group will be some who have been behaviourally inhibited from infancy and who are likely to continue to find school life challenging. Teachers have a range of strategies for helping individual pupils in these groups to settle in and feel more confident. However, long after the majority of pupils have adjusted to their new environment, there will still be a small number of 'reluctant talkers' who are not yet ready to answer oral questions or to participate fully in group discussion. Strategies for encouraging their full participation in the curriculum may include:

- drawing on parents' and carers' knowledge of children's previous patterns of interaction and communication to identify those who may be at risk and need particular attention (e.g. Wolfendale, 1990)
- creating an 'integrative' classroom climate in which cooperation is stressed rather than competition, all pupils are respected whatever their level of performance, and praise is given for supporting others as well as for achieving success oneself
- offering structured as well as unstructured opportunities for group talk (e.g. providing sentence-starters such as 'I wonder how . . . I wish I knew if . . . to encourage question-asking)
- forming groups with the aim of observing their interaction more closely, including a balance of fluent and reluctant talkers so as to ensure that oral work proceeds confidently while those who are having difficulty are presented with successful models but not overwhelmed

- organizing some group work in the classroom in carefully selected pairs rather than larger groups
- making provision for the use of masks, costumes and role play to foster imaginative verbal expression and communication with reduced personal exposure
- monitoring individuals' reactions to more loosely controlled situations such as playtime and movement between activities and provide support and 'tasks' to ease their adjustment to these challenges and divert their attention from sources of intimidation
- ensuring that explicit policies on bullying and harassment, including racial harassment, are understood and followed by all.

                                    (Johnson, 1987; Blatchford and Sharp, 1994;
                                    Jeffries and Dolan, 1994; Chazan et al., 1998).

Some vulnerable children can be helped a great deal through careful advance preparation. Many headteachers and key staff in nurseries and infant schools devote considerable time to their first meetings with parents. Sometimes they will have had information about the child which needs to be discussed. They often suggest that parents visit without the child first to allow an opportunity for them to talk without distraction. Very often this gives parents a chance to voice any worries they have about their child and provides an opening for the teacher to ask a little more. If a child is described as very shy, it is possible to enquire about the situations in which she is most confident speaking, for example whether she is able to speak to people from outside the family who come to the home.

Sometimes a child who is at one of the extremes of the inhibition continuum can benefit from visiting the new setting after school hours when the other children have gone home. The uninhibited child's whirlwind approach causes less disturbance, and it is easier for the parent to deal with it. The child who is extremely behaviourally inhibited finds it easier to explore the nursery in the absence of others and to approach the different activities without freezing. Taking possession of an empty playground when there is no audience makes it easier for him to say, 'I want to go on the horse'. It also allows unobtrusive observation of the level of anxiety the child shows in the new setting.

Where there is still serious concern about the child's ability to settle in, it may next be suggested that the teacher who will be working with him visit him at home before he starts so that he can feel more comfortable with her. We have noted that this is more likely to occur in nurseries and primary schools which have had previous experience with a selectively mute child. The staff find that the benefits of visiting new entry children at home before they start justify the time and effort involved. (See Appendix 1 for notes on home visiting for this purpose.)

Once they begin to attend school, children who are extremely shy and have had little experience in any setting without their mother or extended family need to be confident that they will go home again at the end of the session. It helps if a parent, usually the mother, can stay with them for the first half-day or two so that they know the routine. If a child is still very unhappy and clinging after a few days, it may be necessary to shorten the time they stay there, perhaps coming in for an hour before the end of the morning so that their parent picks them up at the same time as the other children go home. When they can cope with this, it is easy to extend their time in the nursery by 15–30 minutes each day. Some children find reassurance in looking after some small thing that belongs to their mother, perhaps a scarf or gloves, which can be put on a table in their sight as additional proof that she will return.

The child may make a close relationship with one member of staff, with whom he may choose to speak first. It is important that she doesn't become his interpreter and speak for him. ('Andrew would like milk today.') Her relationship with him can be used best in work with him and another quiet child, in games and activities some of which require voiced speech (e.g. a card game such as snap) or which make use of voice-activated toys. Very quiet children are often paired with outgoing talkative children, but working with another quiet but speaking child seems to provide a more encouraging model.

Thus an essential element in prevention is the contribution that teachers can make directly through encouraging quiet children to overcome their inhibitions about talking in school. There is a tendency to 'help' a quiet pupil by speaking for them or addressing them with rhetorical questions that require no answer. Collins (1996) reported that Vicky (aged 10) 'was more likely to talk when I was prepared to be quiet and tolerate the inevitable long silences. Somehow the fact that I was not consciously trying to make her speak allowed her the freedom to speak for herself.' (p. 26) Where specific anxieties play a part in a child's reticence, it may be valuable to acknowledge them and help to put them in perspective or to find practical strategies of dealing with them. Collins (1996, Chapter 8) advocated short programmes of withdrawal work in small groups for habitually quiet pupils, though acknowledging the serious concerns about withdrawal work that many teachers share.

Processes in school which maintain mutism and its effect on teachers and others

Some of the efforts which teachers make to help children settle into school appear actually to have the effect of maintaining and reinforcing selective mutism. Infant teachers are particularly patient about waiting for children to settle. They develop skills in building warm relationships with shy children through encouraging and responding to non-verbal communication. They will use these well-tried and previously successful strategies to help children to relax and communicate, while at the same time looking for opportunities to develop their language skills. Unfortunately this makes it easier for selectively mute children to obtain everything they want without speech (because the teacher's strengths, in effect, reinforce the mutism). For example, Ayllon and Kelly (1974) found that Mona (aged 11) appeared to have all her needs in the classroom met, whether or not they were verbalized.

A child who does not speak receives additional attention. This becomes another factor that maintains the behaviour. Observation of Mona indicated that she was getting more attention for not talking than the other children received for talking. Frequently this status is strengthened by the reaction of other children who also respond to the child's non-verbal demands. When there are visitors to the class, a child will readily explain and confirm the child's silence ('Mary doesn't talk, Miss') (cf. Landgarten, 1975). Very often another child will take on the role of speaking for the selectively mute child.

Sometimes, when a teacher has considerable skill and experience, it is more likely that the early signs of selective mutism will be missed. Because they have enabled many shy children to settle into school gradually, without at first requiring speech from them, they may feel confident that these children too will talk to them in time. Sometimes responding to a child's restricted communication will make the situation worse. Sharon (aged 7) whispered to her teacher when she first went to school and then stopped talking altogether (Crema and Kerr, 1978).

When they look back, teachers are not always sure when they began to be concerned about the child's behaviour. One teacher noticed that the other children no longer expected David (aged 5) to speak and that she was increasingly responding to his non-verbal communication. Retrospectively she remembered that David's behaviour had been odd when he started school: he shut his eyes for the first two days. She found his behaviour difficult to understand because he never seemed to be shy. He was an energetic, highly competitive child whom she described as 'bold', but he was extremely self-conscious if he felt he was being observed and could also be very obstinate. She found this behaviour difficult to understand because it did not fit with her understanding of 'shyness'. When a stereotype of that kind dominates a teacher's thinking, it can obscure the high level of anxiety that a child has about speaking.

After an introductory period with no change, class teachers of mute children will themselves become increasingly anxious. They will be aware that they are making ever increasing efforts to get the mute child to communicate. They will also be concerned with the progress of the child's school work and will be searching for ways to teach which will bypass the refusal to speak. Perhaps the child enjoys being read to and will sometimes point to parts of pictures when asked. These efforts may be double-edged in their effect: they give the children all the opportunities they need to learn and make no demands on them to change

(Edmondson, 1986). Ignoring their silence has no effect. Indeed, it may continue to allow children to avoid situations that make them feel anxious, thus reinforcing the mutism. Whatever the teachers try, they seem to be in a 'no-win' position, and it is easy for them to become preoccupied with the challenge the child presents. A teacher said to one of us: 'Last night I dreamt that Philip spoke to me.'

Some children seem tantalizingly on the point of speaking. Mandy found entry to nursery, primary and secondary schools very difficult. She caused anger and bewilderment when she approached teachers in her early secondary school years, because she gave all the appropriate non-verbal signals that she wanted to say something, but at the last moment she stopped . . . and her teachers felt she deliberately set up this situation. Frustration was also felt by those who taught Gene (aged 14), another child who spoke infrequently (Straughan, 1968). When a teacher persisted in trying to elicit a vocal response from him, he was almost invariably mute and unresponsive. 'When the teacher would eventually give up and move away, he would glance from the corner of his eye at the observers and smile. The observers were unanimous in agreeing that Gene was enjoying a victory.'

The behaviour may precipitate conflict. Sometimes it is felt that there is a hostile quality in the child's silence or behaviour. David once urinated on the classroom floor, apparently because he was refused permission to join a particular activity. His teacher interpreted his behaviour as aggressive, but in the context of classroom rules about not leaving the room without asking for permission, a simpler explanation might have been that he could not leave because he would not ask to do so. This episode illustrates how the children's behaviour can cause conflicting emotions in the adults around them. The anger that is engendered in the teacher may be turned inwards, producing feelings of self-blame. For example, a teacher may speculate that it is her handling of the situation or her reaction to it that is making matters worse (Edmondson, 1986).

Another factor in the situation will be attempts by other teachers to support her. They may be sensitive to her feelings, but at the same time she may be given conflicting advice, for example, to ignore the child's non-verbal communication. This is exceedingly difficult to carry out with consistency, especially as she has responded to it previously. It will also conflict with her wish to teach the child and, in spite of his mutism, to give him all the opportunities offered to the other children in her class.

Unfortunately, the challenge of making a silent child talk is hard for most adults to resist. In the worst scenario other adults will not confine themselves to giving advice but will try out their ideas in a variety of unofficial attempts to make the child speak. A medical student in training, attending a case conference in 1975, was heard to mutter: 'I bet I could make him speak.' In another example from a middle school a headteacher found a class running over the desks. His deputy head who was covering for an absent colleague had meanwhile corralled the selectively mute child into a corner and was beseeching her to speak. It is important to remember that children who adopt this stance will have experienced and resisted many well-intentioned attempts by people outside the family to make them talk long before they come to school, and that each unsuccessful attempt serves to reinforce their behaviour.

Sometimes in the past teachers' frustration with what they saw as the obstinacy of selectively mute children led to numerous uncoordinated attempts by individuals 'to break the child's silence.' These were often promises of prizes for speaking, but as the children were unable to utter a word they never tasted the reward. There might be plans to bribe, trick or trap the child into speaking, but without success. In one classroom, where an 8-year-old boy did not speak for an extended period, the teacher kept him in after school, displayed his name on the board, sent notes to his mother, gave him time-outs of up to 90 minutes and issued him with deadlines by which time he had to speak to her (Watson and Kramer, 1992).

A further effect of the failure of all efforts by the school to help the child was often increasingly negative descriptions of the child and his family by his teachers and a more 'distancing' attitude in meetings with them. The parents would be aware of this, and it would add to their anger and embarrassment over the child's obstinacy and their feelings of resentment and distress about the involvement of other agencies. Today in many cases the negative and damaging features of this account can be avoided, but our discussions with colleagues suggest that each development described here may still occur at times in schools. Selectively mute children do not fit predictable stereotypes and do not respond to conventional methods of management. In school both their teachers and their peers often behave towards them in ways that reinforce their mutism.

Consultation with parents and teachers

Parents

When the difficulties presented by a child like David continue, the teacher will consult the school's special educational needs coordinator (SENCO) and, in smaller schools, the headteacher. In the UK action will be initiated within the framework of the DfES Code of Practice on Special Educational Needs. Initially this will involve collecting all known information about the child and seeking additional information from the parents. Close consultation with them will be expected throughout. It may be helpful at an early stage to have at least one meeting with the parents at which their child is not present. This will make it easier to discuss the child's difficulties sensitively and informally. Teachers will benefit from learning more fully what anxieties the parents share with them about their child and what issues of concern to the school staff have not caused the parents anxiety. They will be able to learn what has been tried in the past and with what result.

A key task will be to list the people to whom the child speaks and in what situations. Here the parents' help is essential, and this process in itself seems to be therapeutic. The parents immediately see the importance of the information they can give, and teachers and other staff are helped to treat them as full partners in the assessment process. This will support them to encourage full communication in a wider range of settings and, if necessary, to collaborate with a teacher or other school staff member in a stimulus fading procedure (see Chapter 7). Participating in this process will also discourage them from fruitless attempts at controlling the child's behaviour through punishment for not speaking or putting the child 'on the spot' to speak in social contexts (Yapko, 2001).

Teachers and other staff

In general, schools and nurseries will not wish to involve external agencies such as an educational psychology service or a speech and language service at an early stage unless it is absolutely necessary. However, when staff are dealing with a situation that is rare and therefore unfamiliar, there may be a case for exploring possible sources of advice and help outside the school sooner rather than later. Initially this may be solely for consultative advice rather than seeking to involve the external specialists in interviewing the child and family. It is important to initiate action to prevent a maladaptive pattern of behaviour becoming entrenched when the child is at nursery or school. (As we noted in Chapter 1, staff in the external services may themselves have little experience of selective mutism. It is helpful if they identify an individual within the team to develop expertise to offer consultation. In one LEA advisory service this function was performed by a teacher who had worked successfully with two selectively mute children in her own classroom in the past. In an educational psychology service a psychologist with a particular interest in relevant approaches to therapy adopted this role. What is crucial is that the individual concerned has the experience to understand the frustration of the school staff and the knowledge to advise on effective helping strategies.)

Within the school a key task for the SENCO will be to communicate what is happening to other members of staff and to explain to them the reasons for discouraging individual 'unofficial' attempts to get the child to speak. Many will not have realized how unsuccessful attempts can make the child more difficult to help. Everyone needs to understand why the programme of intervention must be worked out slowly and carefully to avoid reinforcing what is already a long-established pattern of behaviour. When a strategy is eventually agreed, it will be important that the therapist or psychologist deal with whatever expectations the school staff may hold about the child's treatment. Where will this take place, when will it start, and how long will it go on? What will the consequences of failure be for the child or the teacher? Who will carry responsibility for this, and what will happen next?

But long before that stage is reached, staff will need to have had time to talk about the negative feelings that they may have about the child's refusal to speak. There are likely to be different opinions in the school about the child. A teacher from Essex wrote in 1987: 'Attitudes to K. among the school staff are very mixed. Her teacher wants to help her, but gets very frustrated. The teacher she will go to after Christmas is of the opinion that it is just naughtiness.' Selective mutism gets under teachers' skin. Where it is necessary to reach a consensus on the management of such behaviour across a staff group, meeting time may be needed to air and resolve differences of view.

The first task is to clarify exactly what is happening. It is all too easy for a general statement such as 'She just never talks' to become accepted as the whole truth without adequate checking. Teachers and assistants will find it helpful to pool their observations on the central issues:

- With whom does the child speak, where and under what circumstances, how often, how loudly, with what confidence and fluency, and for how long?
- What are her preferred activities in school?
- Which children does she seek out in the playground, and which adults does she seem to like best?

In fact, it may be difficult for teachers to know how much a child talks to others in the playground. As Buck (1987) pointed out, some selectively mute children will stop an activity when a teacher approaches. Morris (1953) noted that William (aged 7) played with other children, but when observed by a teacher did not speak with them. However, when watched by people other than teachers, he did speak to them. Teaching assistants and other ancillary staff may be able to contribute important observations. Collecting this valuable information is an essential stage in deciding whether an intervention will be possible. The process of describing the behaviour clearly and precisely also helps the teachers to find a different perspective and to regain a sense of optimism about the possibility of change.

The class teacher is likely to find the chance of talking to the teacher of a similar child extremely helpful and reassuring. 'Nobody who hasn't had one can imagine how awful it feels', said a nursery teacher to one of us some years ago. She needs to know enough about the combination of factors which lead to a child not talking in school to realize that it is not simply the result of any failure or mismanagement on her part. For example, Sharon (aged 7) who was described by Crema and Kerr (1978) seemed to have an internal list of people she spoke to and people she did not. She kept to that list very strictly for a long time. Some of the quotations at the beginning of Chapter 1 illustrate how often a teacher feels deskilled and incompetent when faced with a pupil who is persistently mute in school. Contact with others who have known the same feelings may help to reduce the sense of isolation and impotence.

A specific issue that needs to be considered is how the teacher should talk to the child. Sometimes the agreed strategy may be to reduce demands on the child to talk (Tittnich, 1990). Where verbal communication is the focus of attention during an intervention, teachers may find it difficult to alter what have become habitual ways of talking to the child. Rosenbaum and Kellman (1973) made an interesting observation during their intervention. For the first session with the therapist the teacher had prepared several questions which would need a verbal reply. She found this hard 'as she had been so accustomed to phrasing questions which would not require the girl to speak.' A similar comment was made by Straughan whose observations of Mary showed that the teacher used many rhetorical questions when speaking to her. In the normal situation when teachers ask children a question, it is clear that they expect an answer. If an answer is not expected, the question is often asked in a different way: little or no time is given for the reply, and failure to reply is passed over. Rhetorical questions protect the questioner from the embarrassment of no reply, and they allow the other person to remain silent. Many of those who have worked with selectively mute children have noticed a change in their own verbal behaviour: they use many more rhetorical questions and address the child in such a way that no reply is required. Teachers working together may be able to help each other to avoid this.

One of the few detailed accounts of consultative support to school staff who are working with children who are selectively mute was given by Watson (1995) who worked as a speech and language therapist for several sessions a week at a special school for children with moderate learning difficulties. She described the school as very supportive of collaborative and flexible working, and this allowed close liaison with both staff and parents who were keen for her involvement. The child, AJ (aged 10), had attended the school for a number of years and did not speak there at all, or indeed anywhere else outside the family home.

Watson was aware that the staff at the school who had known AJ over an extended period mostly accepted her silence and were good at coping with it. It was going to be important that they change their perceptions and expectations of AJ. They also needed help to know how to react to her and communicate with her as she began to make progress. It was particularly important at each stage that the level of demands made by the staff matched AJ's new level of skill. For example, when she was able to say single words to people, they needed to expect and push for single words, but not more. When she was able to answer questions one to one, the next step was to move towards responding in a small group, but not to expect her to be able to do this when the whole class were present.

It was important too that the staff controlled their reactions when AJ spoke. Her parents confirmed in discussion with Watson that a very calm, low-key response was best. Like many other selectively mute children, she feared that if she did speak there would be a lot of fuss and excitement. Because they knew Watson well, the staff were able to talk about other anxieties, such as making mistakes and 'ruining it all', and how they would feel if they were not one of the 'chosen' people AJ spoke to. Watson covered this through a variety of approaches, including discussion, a written handout and role playing the part of AJ. These covered new ways of interacting with AJ: how much to expect from AJ and in what settings, how to manage if they did not understand what she said and how to respond naturally rather than being distracted by their own nervousness.

Pupils too needed to understand what was happening, so that they knew that although AJ could speak in school, she was still shy and could get upset if her friends tried to get her to say more. Watson was impressed by the sensitivity shown by the pupils, and none of the difficulties that she had anticipated occurred. A fuller account of the work with AJ herself is given in Chapter 8. It extended over 13 school terms and culminated in her successful completion of a work experience placement in a department store and active participation in the choir in the school pantomime – a rare example of successful treatment of a teenager with selective mutism.

When insufficient time is allowed for staff consultation at school, teachers have no opportunity to ensure that the behaviour management regime that is planned is practicable in a classroom setting. Unrelated researchers, one of whom has the same surname, Watson and Kramer (1992), attempted a multi-site intervention to help Tim (aged 8) who had been selectively mute since first learning to speak. The work with the family at home was successful, but the intervention at school was stopped after the first stage. The teachers decided that they could not continue with it 'because of the time and effort involved'. The authors noted in their review of the case that there had been only 3 days between the presentation of the plan by the consulting psychologist and the start of its implementation in the classroom. It appeared that the key teacher who would have to operate the system played no part in designing it, had no background of training or experience with behaviour modification and had no one on whom she could call for support when trying to solve problems that arose as the work proceeded. There is a stark contrast with the support given to school staff in the work with AJ.

Some might contend, however, that it is relatively easy to work with the staff of a small special school. Consultation with the staff of a large secondary school is more complicated, and much depends on the support from members of the senior management team. One of us (SB) has seen how well this can be managed when that support is available. Will, a boy who had not spoken to his teachers in nursery or in two schools at primary level, was due to join a secondary school. Contact with the SENCO at that school was made in the term before he was to start. There had been several unsuccessful attempts to help him, including psychotherapy and a programme of stimulus fading, and it seemed important to make the maximum use of the advantages of a new setting. Because he was extremely anxious the psychiatrist agreed to try medication, starting with a low dose of fluoxetine during the summer holidays. This was gradually increased towards the beginning of term and was carefully monitored.

Preparation in school began before term started with discussions between the parents, the SENCO, a senior learning support assistant (LSA) and a psychologist. In addition, a briefing meeting for all staff who were to teach Will was arranged for the first week of term with a prepared information sheet. This included a brief explanation of selective mutism, a recommended approach for the whole staff and an outline of the initial intervention plan.

The plan was simple and straightforward. Will's mother had previously read with him in one of his primary schools, but this had never been taken forward by arranging for it to be transferred to an LSA or a teacher. It was agreed that from the beginning the LSA (JC) should be established as his key worker at the new school. His mother started reading with him as before, but it was planned with his knowledge and agreement that this would be shortly transferred to a member of staff. Reading took place in a small room away from the classrooms. Will was introduced to JC and agreed that he could read with his mother while she was in the corridor outside. In two stages the key worker moved into the room and took part in the reading. Then his mother was faded out. Other pupils were brought into the sessions. These changed to a game format which was extremely popular and helped to move Will on to using his full voice rather than a loud whisper. Because of his progress his medication was reduced and discontinued shortly after Christmas.

During the next two terms Will spoke during group games to all members of his class, though no group exceeded six children. He read aloud too and answered questions not only from JC but also from another LSA, and also (in JC's presence) his English teacher and his form tutor. This was carried out on different school sites, including the DT and ICT centres, the classroom and the dining hall. It moved on to new targets: 'tell me a joke next time', 'use this to find out the meaning of . . . and tell me . . .', which related both to his school work and his social life with peers. JC was also sensitive to staff feelings of panic or worry about succeeding in their parts in this project and understood the need to extend their confidence in dealing with Will. This was partly achieved by getting teachers to sign a notebook when Will spoke to them, with a reward rate (which he set) of a house point for every five signatures. Importantly, at each stage Will was given a choice of two challenges and always chose the harder one. This confirmed the impression the staff had that he really wanted to speak in school.

During his second year in the school Will continued to receive help from JC, though often indirectly as this was channelled through his teachers. He found it hard to assert himself in a group, but developed a wide range of interests in and out of school, running a quiet games club during the lunch hour. Will is an intelligent boy who has been fortunate in the support and understanding he has had from his parents and teachers. However, they would agree that, although he is now a confident speaker in most situations, he will always be socially anxious and can still experience stress and discomfort which can inhibit him from using his full voice. It is hoped to start a social skills group based in the school for pupils with social anxiety and similar difficulties. This underlines the need for continued help for children who have been selectively mute as they move into adolescence.

Teachers who are interested in managing speech anxiety in everyday situations in such a way as to facilitate speech will find a useful list of suggestions in Johnson and Wintgens' *Selective Mutism Resource Manual* (2001, pp. 95–103). A short account of the strategies they favour is given here in Chapter 8.

Interventions based in school

Use of reinforcement and stimulus fading

A number of case studies describe interventions carried out entirely or almost entirely in school. The interventions commonly use stimulus fading (see Chapter 6), often in combination with other behavioural techniques. Richards and Hansen (1978) provide an excellent example of a programme carried out with Amy (aged 8) by her classroom teacher. This started in a situation where Amy always spoke (home) and gradually moved to a situation where she had never spoken (school with the teacher and the whole class present). The different dimensions of difficulty for Amy included place (e.g. the route to school, the playground, the classroom), the number of children present, the difficulty of the verbal response required and its volume and frequency. The criterion for success and reward varied for each session, but always demanded improvement on at least one dimension. The authors point out the need to pay attention to school politics in setting up an intervention in school by obtaining permission and cooperation from all the school staff beforehand.

Hill and Scull (1985) worked with a boy who was a reluctant speaker rather than selectively mute. His problems included a generally low level of activity in addition to his infrequent speech. The professionals in the residential school where Mark was placed learned a great deal from the way his mother played with him on her visits. When she played games with him and asked a question, she immediately shifted her attention away from him and took up another activity until he answered. The staff modified the rules of some games so that the players had to speak or call out to get a turn. If Mark did not speak, he missed a turn, and the game continued whether or not he spoke (for a more detailed account, see below). It was not easy for the staff, including the authors, to apply these strategies consistently. They observe that in teaching and in most forms of therapy, the usual approach is for teachers to adjust their behaviour to the client's responses and to pace progress according to the feedback from what the client does. In Mark's case, this had led to prolonged waiting with no response in the end. Mark's treatment helped him to speak more often, to participate in class and to begin to learn in all basic subjects. However, he continued to have some physical difficulties and to be a slow responder who seldom initiated new activities. The authors emphasize how hard it was for staff to abandon principles of treatment and teaching that had worked well with other children.

Richards and Hansen used Amy's home as a starting point for a school-based programme. In Hill and Scull's study the therapists observed and used the mother's strategies. In the case study by Crema and Kerr (1978) the first attempt at intervention failed, using a school-based programme which combined escape/avoidance while ignoring mute behaviour and rewarding speech. Sharon was isolated from the class behind a partition and given nothing to do all day unless she said a key word at certain times which would allow her to take part in the class activity. The programme failed to produce speech from Sharon and had to be abandoned because of the deterioration in her behaviour at home. The therapists felt that Sharon's father had sabotaged the programme by saying in her hearing that it would not succeed. With hindsight, it is easy to see that the intervention programme gave Sharon little chance of obtaining a reward, placed her in a situation where she felt most anxious about speaking and demanded a level of response that was not possible for her in that situation. Success was obtained eventually, after Sharon had been moved to a residential setting. The intervention there involved an intensive and complex programme with an emphasis on positive reinforcement. Nine months later Sharon was able to return to her old school after workers from the residential school had provided two sessions of training to build up the staff's confidence and 'overcome their apprehension and scepticism about her return.' The length of time that was taken and the number of stages needed to complete the intervention should warn us against trying the same approach in a school setting. The original approach was based on response cost (which punishes the child for not responding). This is likely to increase the child's level of anxiety and jeopardize the parents' support.

Croghan and Craven (1982) review the lengthy course of the various interventions with JB (aged 8) which extended over a 5-year period. The initial approach was to try to change her mute behaviour through external reinforcement in the school setting. Early failure was overcome when the therapists recognized JB's high level of anxiety and used different techniques (see Chapter 6). But they reflected that success could have been achieved much more quickly and with less pain if they had studied the child's history more carefully and noted the natural reinforcing agents who were available within her own family. They (the family) showed the way when they used a form of stimulus fading, playing games with her mother and brother to 'fade in' her new stepfather. It is essential to use every possible source of information about what will act as a natural reinforcer for a selectively mute child. Often teachers have been able helpfully to suggest a wide variety of activities which might be effective sources of reinforcement for particular children, as have parents and children themselves. The range of possibilities is very great. For example, Lazarus, Gavillo and Moore (1983) mention bubble blowing, talking to the classroom rabbit and the use of puppets in just two case studies.

One of us (SB) remembers a nursery child, a girl of nearly 4. Sonia was referred by an experienced and sensitive headteacher because she had not spoken at all in the first 6 weeks in the nursery and was increasingly passive and inactive. On a home visit her mother explained that she had had similar problems as a child and that this made her particularly anxious about her daughter's difficulties. She found herself beginning to weep when she had to leave Sonia crying at the nursery. We spoke about the little girl's special interests and at that point she asked her daughter to come in with 'the bird'. The psychologist expected something like a budgerigar, but the child came in carrying an enormous and extremely beautiful cockatiel. We admired him in silence. Finally the psychologist asked what he was called. 'His name is Gilbert,' she said, and continued to talk about him. We wondered if he would like to visit the nursery. Of course, the headteacher agreed. Gilbert was a success as a visitor, and his owner made rapid progress in confident speaking. From then on, in that nursery, making home visits was known as 'bringing the cockatiel to school'.

Use of peers in school-based programmes

The peer group can be a major resource for work with selectively mute children in school. In a typical programme Calhoun and Koenig (1973) worked with the teachers of four children aged 5–8. They introduced operant procedures to the teachers on an individual basis and reached agreement through joint planning on reinforcement procedures in which the whole class obtained rewards for increased speaking by the target child. This avoided further isolation of the children (e.g. through behavioural treatment in a withdrawal room). It also ensured peer approval for their attempts to speak, which might otherwise have sometimes been ignored.

Working with Mary (aged 15) Straughan (1968) also made it possible for the other pupils in Mary's special class to obtain rewards from the intervention. In this case use was made of a signal light which could easily be turned on and off. A period of 25 minutes every day was designated as the treatment session. During this period each time that Mary spoke, the signal light was turned on, and the event was recorded. When the light came on, she earned points which contributed to the size of rewards (initially candies and later other gifts) that were to be shared by Mary with the whole class. It was important that the other children were reminded not to respond to Mary's non-verbal communication. Each day the amount she had earned for the class was announced. After reluctance on the first day she was described as 'very happy with the procedure and extremely fond of sharing the candy with the class'. Her frequency of talking in that class increased, and her peers' behaviour towards her changed. Her mother also reported that she began to talk a little more freely at home. However, within school the increase in Mary's talking was specific to that situation only and did not generalize to her behaviour in other classes.

Winter (1984) used four children as peer therapists to increase the frequency of Neil's speech. All the children were pupils in a language unit attached to a primary school. Neil (aged 7) was making very little progress and spent much of his day playing alone. The staff had noticed that the other children no longer expected Neil to speak and seldom spoke to him, though they often spoke for him. The programme was agreed with staff and then explained to Neil and the four other children. Each time he spoke to an adult or one of the peer therapists, they would give him a token which could be exchanged later for a sweet (candy). In addition, praise and positive feedback were also given, and extra activities to encourage speech were set up. Staff were asked to ignore Neil's silence by walking away if he refused to answer. Before the programme started Neil was shown how to exchange the tokens for sweets. There were some initial difficulties: 'The peer therapists were not consistent enough, and staff were not vigilant enough in monitoring the peer therapists' performance. In addition, the back-up reinforcer (chosen by the headteacher) was grossly inappropriate, being a rather large strawberry-shaped 'gobstopper' which effectively prevented Neil speaking for several minutes afterwards!' Discussion, video feedback and a change of back-up (to smaller sweets) overcame these problems. The intervention began to be effective, and after 4 weeks Neil was speaking spontaneously, even to new visitors.

Ciottone and Madonna (1984) introduced William, an 11-year-old boy who had been almost entirely silent at school since first grade, into a small weekly group with two other boys. They met, together with the school counsellor, once a week for 45 minutes over 20 sessions. William was never ridiculed by his peers in the group, but on several occasions they made statements about his non-verbal behaviour that caused him some anxiety and thus 'served to upset in a productive way his reliance on a dysfunctional interactive pattern' (p. 26). They sometimes used video equipment to role-play interview situations in which the counsellor acted as a roving reporter. The turning point in William's progress came when he grabbed the microphone from the counsellor one day and took on the role of interviewer himself. An important step towards the generalization of new patterns of communication to other settings came from group excursions in which they visited various parts of the school and from visits by one of his teachers to the group setting. A similar use of what these authors called a 'transitional object' has been reported by many authors concerned with the treatment of selective mutism. We will discuss the concept of 'stimulus fading' in Chapter 7.

Other examples of the use of peers in school-based intervention are reported by Conrad, Delk and Williams (1974) and Clayton (1981), whose case studies are described in Chapter 6. For another report of a case intervention involving a school counsellor see Richburg and Cobia (1994).

Interventions using reading tasks and simple audio recording

School-based interventions are facilitated if they focus on behaviour that occurs naturally in that setting and is what is expected there. Everyone knows that school is a place where a child learns to read. Looking at a book and 'speaking' to it rather than to an adult is often less threatening for a selectively mute child, so reading tasks have often featured in intervention programmes for selective mutism in school. For example, Scott (1977) used a reading task in a graded programme of desensitization with Linda (aged 6). This was built around the one positive observation that Linda was able to read in school if she was able to use a tape-recorder alone in a quiet room. A number of different adults were introduced in this safe setting before Linda was able to transfer her new skills successfully to the classroom. Scott's case study is described in more detail in Chapter 6.

Rosenbaum and Kellman (1973) also used reading to help a 9-year-old girl who was still mute in school after 3 years of attendance. She was the daughter of a Brazilian family living in Wisconsin. Her parents were unhappy with the school and had rejected suggestions that she be referred for outside help. However, she did begin to speak with a speech therapist in a one-to-one session in school. Some of the sessions when she read aloud to the therapist were recorded, and the girl then took the tape to her class teacher who played them to the child's reading group in her presence. 'This was the first time the teacher had heard her voice.' The teacher was then faded in (see Chapters 5 and 6) to one session with the therapist and took part in a conversation which continued as she and the child walked back to the empty classroom. There were three children in her class who were also in the reading group and had therefore heard the tape. In the next step they were added to the therapist's sessions, one at a time.

Following this, the child was asked to invite four other children from her class to the therapist's sessions. 'The children considered it a privilege to be invited to a session, and (she) was proud to do the inviting.' This continued for 10 weeks until all the children from the class had had a turn, and the child was beginning to respond to questions in front of the whole class. Important points in the success of this intervention were the child's control over the use of the tape and the status she acquired in selecting the children to invite. Her status in the classroom had been that of a girl for whom peers would cover by answering questions for her. That status was now transformed. This may have been as important in enabling her to maintain and generalize her gains as was the fine grading of the steps in the programme in the first place in enabling her to start speaking.

Books and tape-recorders are not the only objects that can mediate a potentially threatening communication so that the child does not face the listener directly as he or she speaks. Other workers have successfully used puppets (Kelly, 1981), a toy telephone (Kass et al., 1967; Heimlich, 1981), a real telephone (Sluckin, 1977), and a book for home–school communication (Southworth, 1988). It seems likely that computer games will soon be added to this list, as they become fully established. There is the potential to set up a situation in which a child speaks about a game while looking at the computer screen rather than at the person who is being addressed. (See also the section 'Adjuncts to therapy' in Chapter 8.)

Use of audio and video recording to foster children's perception of their own competence

Another technique for helping selective mutes which has been based in schools is self-modelling. This uses video recording of the teacher asking questions in the child's classroom. Recordings are also made using family members to whom the child speaks freely. In these recordings family members put to the child the same questions that were put by the teacher in the classroom. This time the child will give oral answers. The two recordings are then edited together to produce a fake video in which the child appears to answer questions competently in the classroom. This is shown several times to the child. Dowrick and Hood (1978), Pigott and Gonzales (1987) and Kehle, Owen and Cressy (1990) have used this type of intervention with success. Its rationale (see Chapter 6) comes from social learning theory, which would predict that self-modelling will help these children to speak because it changes their perception of their own effectiveness. There have been attempts to change the behaviour through peer modelling rather than self-modelling, but these are predicted to have less effect, as they will show up the children's incompetence in comparison with normally speaking peers (Dowrick, 1983).

This approach has a convincing theoretical basis, and the reported success rate is high. It might have been expected that it would be widely adopted and developed further. But the process is a lengthy one, and the technical equipment and expertise are not often easily available to those involved in planning treatment for selectively mute children. Holmbeck and Lavigne (1992) devised a variant on the strategy which eliminated the need for videotape editing. They followed through a stimulus fading process and shot a series of video sequences in which their selectively mute client, Mary, was initially speaking with her mother and eventually speaking with the therapist. 'After talking was established at each step, videotape feedback was employed both as a self-modelling technique and as a reinforcer' (p. 665).

Blum et al. (1998) used audiotape instead of videotapes. They reported on three girls aged 6–9 years who had not responded to previous attempts at intervention and who not only started speaking very soon to the individuals who featured in the audiotape but also generalized that behaviour to other people to whom they had not talked previously. This technique offers great promise, and a simple guide to it is given in Appendix 3. An audiotape is much easier to make for this purpose than a videotape, because the process is simpler, the technology is more widely available and it is not necessary to match background scenery in the two parts of the tape. But there are no panaceas: Blum and his colleagues report that three other children refused to participate in making a tape and two children who did make a tape did not begin to answer questions after listening to their tape. Perhaps longer tapes, or a schedule in which children listen to the tape more frequently, might be more effective in a wider range of cases. They also speculated that 'seeing and hearing oneself speak may be more effective than just hearing oneself speak' (p. 43). However, a dubbed audiotape played a part in the successful intervention described by Powell and Dalley (1995). Further research on these approaches is needed in order to identify the key factors that are associated with successful outcomes.

A similar theoretical position underpinned the analysis by Lachenmeyer and Gibbs (1985) of the social-psychological functions of reward. Their theoretical argument has practical implications. They highlight the different functions that reward can have and emphasize its value as social feedback on performance. When managed well, it will encourage children to attribute success to their own efforts and increase their feeling of competence. Children should increasingly be involved in setting up reward contingencies themselves, and when possible, these should represent choice rather than compulsion. Lachenmeyer and Gibbs applied the principle in intervention with Joey (aged 4) who had not spoken outside his family for the 18 months he had been in a nursery. In fact he had spoken just once – when a teacher who was new to the school asked him during a limbo game whether he wanted the bar to go up or down. Key features in the situation that might have facilitated his giving an answer appeared to be that the teacher was new, that the question only needed an easy one-word response, and that giving that response gained him control over an activity which he enjoyed. His teacher was asked to withdraw him to play games which he enjoyed, provided that he gave a brief answer. In time this led to longer responses to the teacher, and then to speech in front of other children. This was extended to other social situations, starting from rewards for simple new responses. Eventually the control of rewards was put under Joey's control: his mother gave him a sweet if he told her that he had spoken in situations where she had not been present. This shift was intended to stress the 'feedback' component of reward and 'to maximize his awareness of his own success and competence'. A similar procedure was used in work with an older child by Beck and Hubbard (1987). Her teacher helped her to keep a list of people she had spoken to. At regular intervals she was encouraged to select the next person to add to the list. As noted in Chapter 2, selectively mute children often manifest a strong need to control others. At the same time they also show anxiety about speaking in some settings. There is much to be said for behavioural strategies that offer them a degree of control and sustain their sense of their own competence.

Effect of selective mutism on children's learning

Talk between pupils and teachers and talk among pupils plays a crucial role in children's learning at school. Teachers rely on what they hear pupils say in order to assess and support their learning. For that reason Collins (1996) argued that it is important that pupils are 'active participants in the discourse of the classroom' (p. 2). If they do not participate, they will be prevented from learning to express themselves, from asking questions and making the learning their own and from exploring the theme of a lesson actively. Non-participation may affect their self-image in a negative way, may lead to social isolation and may make them vulnerable to bullying (p. 9). Similar arguments were put forward by Jeffries and Dolan (1994) who describe talking in the classroom as 'one of the major means by which enquiry can be conducted . . . an essential tool for learning in every area of the curriculum' (p. 117).

Some aspects of this wide-ranging concern about quiet pupils are not entirely supported by the available evidence on the educational progress of selectively mute children. For example, nearly 70% of those who were identified in the Finnish survey by Kumpulainen et al. (1998) were reported by their teachers to be performing at or above the average level for their group in school. This raises questions about the best way to treat a child who is making good progress with most school work but does not speak. (The issue of whether therapeutic intervention is justified is discussed in the next section.) How far should teachers accommodate to the children's wish to learn by responding to their non-verbal signals? Conversely, how consistently can teachers ignore the non-verbal communication and still satisfy the wish to teach them? Many selectively mute children will participate fully in all classroom activities except those that require speaking. For example, William (aged 10) managed competently in all areas except oral work. This even extended sometimes to volunteering to do blackboard exercises (Bednar 1974). Similarly Elson et al. (1965) described the case of a girl who did well with her written work at school, but refused to read aloud or recite.

Some children appear to have suffered educationally. For example, Hayden (1980) suggested that Kevin had to repeat a year 'because he did not talk to teachers and no-one knew whether or not he was learning'. Adams (1970) described a child who had to repeat first grade although his written work had been done, because of the lack of oral work. Emma (aged 6) who was described by Wulbert et al. (1973) was an extremely passive pupil. 'Although she lived just across the street from the school and played actively there, she had only to cross the street to become a pliable mannequin. In addition to not speaking, Emma never participated in any motor activities. She carried home the school craft materials, and made at home the things that the others had made in class. She eagerly related to her mother all that went on in school each day . . .' A very similar description is given of Eric (aged 6) by Morin, Ladouceur and Cloutier (1982). However, it is impossible to generalize about the academic achievement of children with selective mutism. As Stone et al. (2002) pointed out, researchers have rarely studied academic progress over the course of treatment, even in detailed qualitative case studies. The issue has also been ignored in most of the recent surveys of larger groups of children, with the exception of the Finnish study mentioned above.

Many teachers have found ingenious ways of teaching and testing a selectively mute child's reading. For example, David, who was described above, evidently wished to learn to read. So his teacher changed her normal practice of listening to children read aloud to her. When he brought his book to her and pointed to a word she supplied it at once. At the end of the book, when she checked his words, he pointed to each word as she said it. Other teachers have worked closely with parents on tape recording their children's reading. The child will take a book home and record themselves reading it. The next day they will give or play the recording to the teacher with the book in front of them.

Earlier in the chapter, we noted the value of reading into an audio recorder in school as a task that approximates to normal verbal communication and can be used as a step towards talking. The use of an audio recorder in school may also simply be used as a medium for learning. Scott (1977) whose work was mentioned earlier provides an example of this:

Linda's educational attainment was congruent with her ability in that she prepared her reading appropriate to her age level with her mother and seemed to benefit fully from classroom activities. She appeared to be an intelligent child. On the Wechsler Intelligence Scale for Children performance scale she scored 124. She was encouraged to do her reading alone on to a cassette tape-recorder in a quiet room in school. This was a successful venture and the practice was maintained.

Up to this point we have taken a positive view of the children's ability to learn in school in spite of their refusal to speak. Such a view can only be maintained as long as one concentrates on the written curriculum. It is no accident that the examples that were quoted all involved activities such as reading where the child focuses on an object such as a book or a piece of craft work rather than on another person. But a social dimension is a central feature of modern versions of the school curriculum. Even an overtly 'traditional' framework such as the National Curriculum in England emphasizes educational objectives relating to interpersonal and social skills. Thus the Statutory Order for the curriculum for English (DfES, 2000) requires that 'teaching should ensure that work in speaking and listening, reading and writing is integrated'. During Key Stage 1 (aged 5–7) the overriding aim of work on speaking is that pupils should learn to 'speak clearly, fluently and confidently to different people'. Specifically they 'should be taught to:

- speak with clear diction and appropriate intonation
- choose words with precision
- organize what they say
- focus on the main point(s)
- include relevant detail
- take into account the needs of their listeners'

The learning context should enable them to 'learn to speak clearly, thinking about the needs of their listeners. They work in small groups and as a class, joining in discussions and making relevant points. They also learn how to listen carefully to what other people are saying, so that they can remember the main points. They learn to use language in imaginative ways and express their ideas and feelings when working in role and in drama activities.'

During Key Stage 2 (aged 8–11) the overriding aim of work on speaking is that pupils should learn to 'speak with confidence in a range of contexts, adapting their speech for a range of purposes and audiences'. Specifically they 'should be taught to:

- use vocabulary and syntax that enables them to communicate more complex meanings
- gain and maintain the interest and response of different audiences [for example, by exaggeration, humour, varying pace and using persuasive language to achieve particular effects]

- choose material that is relevant to the topic and to the listeners
- show clear shape and organization with an introduction and an ending
- speak audibly and clearly, using spoken standard English in formal contexts
- evaluate their speech and reflect on how it varies'

The learning context should enable them to 'learn how to speak in a range of contexts, adapting what they say and how they say it to the purpose and the audience. Taking varied roles in groups gives them opportunities to contribute to situations with different demands. They also learn to respond appropriately to others, thinking about what has been said and the language used.'

During Key Stages 3–4 (aged 11–16) the overriding aim of work on speaking is that pupils should learn to 'speak fluently and appropriately in different contexts, adapting their talk for a range of purposes and audiences, including the more formal'. Specifically they 'should be taught to:

- structure their talk clearly, using markers so that their listeners can follow the line of thought
- use illustrations, evidence and anecdote to enrich and explain their ideas
- use gesture, tone, pace and rhetorical devices for emphasis
- use visual aids and images to enhance communication
- vary word choices, including technical vocabulary and sentence structure, for different audiences
- use spoken standard English fluently in different contexts
- evaluate the effectiveness of their speech and consider how to adapt it to a range of situations'

The learning context should enable them to 'learn to speak and listen confidently in a wide variety of contexts. They learn to be flexible, adapting what they say and how they say it to different situations and people. When they speak formally or to people they do not know, they are articulate and fluent in their use of spoken standard English. They learn how to evaluate the contributions they, and others, have made to discussions and drama activities. They take leading and other roles in group work.' (The Statutory Orders may be examined at http://www.nc.uk.net)

Reflecting international trends, education reforms in the UK have made a broad and balanced curriculum a statutory entitlement for every child. The challenge to the non-speaking child is not restricted to English. Various attainment targets in the other core subjects and in foundation subjects also involve a social dimension. Ideas and questions are discussed in whole class or smaller class groups, and reports may take many different forms, including giving an oral report to the rest of the class. Their speaking skills are crucial to the achievement of the full learning objectives. For example, in Design and Technology in Year 4 (aged 9–10) there is a unit called 'Lighting it up'.

In this unit, children apply knowledge about electric circuits that they have acquired in science in a purposeful way. They learn to design and make something that will shine light, e.g. a table lamp, a light in a room, or one that lights up a poster, a Christmas tree or a display. The children will also need to consider what kind of lights are switched on and off by remote control, e.g. in a corridor or in a home so that it looks lived in. While many of the designing and making skills will be used, there will be two particular focuses. The children should be encouraged to define a set of clear specifications for the light by considering who will use it, and the conditions under which it might be used. They may also use ICT tools to support their research into a range of lights and to control their light, switching it on and off when required.

(See http://www.standards.dfes.gov.uk/schemes/designtech)

There have been radical changes in the curriculum since Smayling (1959) could write of a very bright selectively mute 10-year-old: 'On school achievement tests he scored highest consistently in his classroom and frequently scored highest in school.' Now, unless children achieve the social objectives of the curriculum, it will not be possible to claim that they are meeting the basic requirements of school learning.

The message that contributions to oral work really are important can be conveyed by involving pupils in assessing their own contributions themselves. Collins (1996) reported the following list of self-assessment questions that emerged from a series of class discussions on the topic:

- How well did I try to include others?
- How well did I listen to other people's ideas?
- How well did I express my feelings?
- How well did I share my feelings?
- How well did I show respect for other people's ideas and feelings?
- Did I ask questions?
- Did I use an appropriate level of voice?
- Did I disagree with other people without putting them down? (p. 161)

She had pupils rate each aspect of their contribution to specific lessons on a five-point scale and found that this helped them to learn over time what was expected of them.

In spite of their problems in relating to adults, selectively mute children often enjoy fairly successful relationships with some of their peers in school. Teachers have shown ingenuity in developing strategies to enable a selectively mute child to participate in shared and group activities in the classroom. One example noted above was the work of Hill and Scull (1985) with Mark (aged 9+), adapting strategies his mother had developed for making it easy for him to speak.

First, the rules of familiar games were modified so that participants had to speak (e.g. call out a name, ask for a card, count, answer a question) before taking a turn. If Mark did not speak he missed his turn. Whether or not he spoke, the game continued. As his skill at responding and reading ability progressed, he became able to read recipes, math flash cards, and riddles out loud when they were presented in game-like format. Second, a small-group question-answering activity was developed. When Mark was asked a question, he was told to whisper the answer to the child beside him when he was ready. The teacher then immediately shifted attention from him by asking another child a question. In this way Mark was usually able to whisper answers to other children and sometimes call out his answer to the group.

This example illustrates the point that any attempt to offer a full education to a selectively mute child ultimately involves what all teachers instinctively expect – working towards relaxed and confident speech in the classroom. Yet some authors have argued against early intervention in these cases, suggesting that more harm than good may be done if the intervention goes wrong and that adults' impatience to have the child talking is motivated more by their own frustration than by a selfless concern for the good of the child. The arguments for and against intervention and the question of timing an intervention for the best chances of success are explored in the next two sections.

Arguments for and against intervention

'Our initial and emphatic advice to a school or teacher faced with a child who persistently behaves in this way is to think first not about what to do but whether to take any action at all. It seems reasonable to us that any intervention should have a clear and justified basis such as would be provided by evidence that the future development of that child and/or his peers would be impaired if no action were taken.' Lumb and Wolf (1988), who presented this challenge, asserted that such evidence is extremely hard to find. Specifically they claimed that:

• Many of the children show normal social and occupational adjustment when followed up into adulthood 'regardless of whether "treatment" in childhood had succeeded'.
• There is no evidence that other children are adversely affected.
• Many of the interventions that have been carried have been 'intrusive and disruptive'.

We agree with Lumb and Wolff's second point but do not in any case regard effects on other children as a significant reason for intervening in selective mutism. As will appear in later chapters, we also agree with their third point. Indeed, a small number of reported interventions have been worse than intrusive. It is not unreasonable to suggest that one or two of those involving aversive strategies have verged on the cruel (e.g. Van der Kooy and Webster, 1975). But the fact that some methods of intervention have been intrusive or disruptive does not mean that all methods need to be. The strategies outlined in Chapters 7 and 8 are designed to enable those planning an intervention to choose the least intrusive method that will meet the needs of the situation.

We cannot agree with Lumb and Wolff's first point. There have been very few long-term follow-up studies of selectively mute children (see Chapter 9). Some of those that have shown disappointing results relate to interventions of an unsatisfactory kind involving hospitalization with unspecified treatment (e.g. Koch and Goodlund, 1973; Wergeland, 1979). In the latter study none of the treated children received any form of behaviour therapy. On the other hand, when Reed (1963) followed up four young adults who had been seen earlier at a community child guidance clinic, those whose social adjustment was described most positively were those whose clinic treatment had appeared most successful at the time. We have not been able to trace any published reports other than Wergeland's that followed up untreated children into adulthood. Nor is it yet possible to find published reports of the adult outcomes of recent innovations in behavioural methods of intervention.

There is a further cause for concern if a decision is made not to intervene. The situation in which the child is placed is dynamic. Non-intervention by one group of workers will not prevent others officially or unofficially trying to elicit speech from the child. Many find it hard to resist the temptation to show their professional skill and achieve a breakthrough where others have been unsuccessful. It is better to intervene in a planned and minimally intrusive way than to risk developing a further overlay of resistance in the child as a result of confused and uncoordinated efforts.

Powell and Dalley (1995) argued that the key factor in a decision to intervene should be the impact of selective mutism on aspects of child development such as the ability to engage fully in social and educational interactions at school. The 6-year-old girl with whom they were concerned was actively involved in school activities and making progress in academic learning, but she was not participating fully in all aspects of classroom life such as plays, songs and oral discussion. A particular influence on their commitment to her treatment was that she repeatedly made clear to her parents at home that she really wanted to speak at school.

There is some evidence that the immediate and short-term outcome is more favourable when children receive help at an early stage. In a follow-up of 24 children Kolvin and Fundudis (1981) found that when marked improvement occurred it did so before the child reached the age of 10. Those children who had failed to improve by this age were much less likely to do so later. In another follow-up study with the same number of children Wright (1968) found that they had 'responded well to short-term treatment, particularly when they were referred at an early age'. Nash et al. (1979) reached the same conclusion after reviewing work with smaller numbers of children. They commented that 'early intervention had the advantage of preventing secondary deficits and other harmful effects upon the children's learning'. Similar arguments are presented by Austad, Sininger and Stricken (1980), Wright et al. (1985), Porjes (1992), Holmbeck and Lavigne (1992) and Imich (1998). Some investigators have reported that children's academic performance improved significantly after they had overcome selective mutism (e.g. Giddan et al., 1997). The only systematic quantitative review of the effectiveness of treatment in selective mutism has indicated that, when treatment is begun within a shorter time interval after its onset, there are better results (Stone et al., 2002).

There is no doubt that mutism may become very much more difficult to treat when there is a very long delay before intervention or when unsuccessful interventions increase a young person's resistance. As noted in Chapter 2, young people in their teens who have been selectively mute for a number of years sometimes present a picture of complex and deep-seated emotional disturbance with a wide range of deviant behaviour patterns (Youngerman, 1979; Hayden, 1980; Roberts, 1984; Tibbles and Russell, 1992). It appears from the literature that simple and positive forms of intervention may have a higher chance of success with younger children. (See discussion of escape/avoidance strategies in Chapter 7.)

Thus the balance of the available evidence seems to favour early intervention and offers little support for a non-interventionist position. A strong argument for early intervention is that it can be carried out with a light touch, often using the parents as co-workers to establish speech in settings other than the home. An additional advantage is that early intervention can be planned before the child starts school where there are so many factors that will reinforce non-verbal communication.

Without early intervention the behaviour becomes entrenched because being silent brings rewards:

- Mutism is negatively reinforced because not speaking relieves anxiety, and gets attention (and special treatment).
- Non-verbal communication gets what you want and is positively reinforced.
- Not speaking avoids the upsetting psychological sequelae.
- There is no reason to change established behaviour which is comfortable.

Lumb and Wolff emphasized how upset and frustrated most adults become when working with a selectively mute child. Perhaps intervention would 'reflect the needs of parents and teachers rather than the needs of the child'. The urge to take action could lead to unnecessary or excessive interventions. It is not possible to identify any research evidence bearing on this point, but the possibility cannot be dismissed out of hand. There is at least a risk that anger and frustration might 'distort perceptions of what is happening' and lead to an excessive response. We consider that the most convincing safeguards against this will be a full awareness of the danger and a confident grasp of what a 'least intrusive' intervention could involve.

Timing of intervention in relation to events in school

The timing of intervention involves other considerations besides age. It is possible to time a school-related intervention to make maximum use of rhythms of change that are built into the normal school year. The starting point for this is the observation that some children will begin to talk when they have a new teacher or move to a new school. There have been many illustrations of this in the literature (e.g. Brison, 1966; Bozigar and Hansen, 1984). Wergeland (1979) described a group of young people who only began to talk when they left school and moved away to work, but who remained mute when they met people who had known them in the days when they did not talk. It seems that some children and young people who are ready to talk find it difficult to do so with those to whom they have refused to speak in the past. So, for some children at least, the optimum time for intervention may be when they move to a new class (preferably with advance preparation of those involved – see the account of Will above). It is interesting to note that some successful interventions employing new techniques have capitalized on this. For example, one of the earliest reports of a successful intervention through drug therapy alone described treatment that began when a 12-year-old girl started her school summer vacation and was judged successful when she returned for the new school year and 'spoke freely with adults and peers' (Black and Uhde, 1992, p. 1091).

As we have suggested elsewhere, this timing may be distressing for the previous class teacher who may have been responsible for highlighting the need for help in the first place (Baldwin and Cline, 1991). If this teacher can understand the influence of the setting on speaking and not speaking, it will be easier for her to appreciate the advantages of this timing. Both the teachers should be involved in the planning of a strategy along these lines. After all, it is counter-intuitive: most people would expect children to find it easier to start speaking in a setting that is familiar to them.

It would be wrong to suggest that a change of either class or school in itself is enough to effect a change in the behaviour of most of the children. Wright (1968) reported that, when a change of class was arranged for several children 'because of apparent conflict between child and teacher', it did not have a positive result. Bozigar and Hansen (1984) stressed that the successful school transfers that were arranged for the four children in their group had their effect because of the earlier investment in group psychotherapy. Then the change to a different school secured each child's 'new role as a verbal member of her class and of society'. In relation to the timing of intervention, as to many other features of work with selectively mute children, action at one level or of one kind is not enough on its own. What most of the children require is a multi-level approach in which their school works in partnership with another agency and with their parents to secure change across different settings. The detail of what that approach might be is the subject of later chapters.

Chapter 5
The development of non-behavioural approaches: a historical review

The history of treatments for selective mutism mirrors the history of psychological treatment generally. In his classic paper on the concept of selective mutism Tramer gave an unusual report of therapeutic success: sudden improvement after beginning to wear 'blessed wax' sewn into a waistcoat. Those who have encountered the unusual and disturbing patterns of behaviour associated with selective mutism will sympathize with the desire for a miracle cure. The common-sense methods that some professionals adopted initially had little success. Many authors have reaffirmed the futility of cursory advice, admonitions and exhortations (e.g. Reed, 1963; Elson et al., 1965; Wergeland, 1979). The recognition of this truism has not always been constructive. Describing the refusal to speak by Rex (aged 3) Rigby (1929) affirmed that 'soft words and coaxing' would not suffice and went on to advocate 'military discipline' as the quickest strategy. 'He may exhaust the disciplinarian in a few hours but he must be attacked at the moment when he himself is worn out and there must be no relaxing of the rule. It will be a long task and a hard one, but only when this boy is obedient will he be rescued from imbecility.'

At a later stage of the history of child psychotherapy conventional therapists continued to find selective mutism particularly difficult to treat. There are frequent comments in the literature on the exceptional problems it presents, the length of time it takes, the frustrations therapists experience, and the low rate of success. For example, Kolvin and Fundudis (1981) found that less than half of their sample of 24 treated cases had improved significantly when followed up after 5–10 years. Explanations vary as to why these approaches to treatment tended to have such a poor outcome. One reason may be that the symptom is often very strongly established before the child is referred for help (Wright, 1968). Many accounts highlight a second possible reason – the fact that this simple-seeming phenomenon is psychologically very complex. From a psychoanalytic perspective Radford (1977) concluded a report of a long and very difficult treatment case by emphasizing 'the complexity of the many internal and external factors seemingly involved'. Working within a different framework Reed (1963) argued that, because selective mutism develops in a variety of ways, it would be impossible to find a single standard effective therapeutic procedure.

Historically the earliest systematic attempts at intervention in selective mutism were in the psychodynamic tradition. As noted in Chapter 2, there was little consensus among psychodynamic writers about the origins and development of this pattern of symptoms. Equally, as Kratochwill (1981) pointed out after a detailed review, there was little evidence of a steadily growing expertise in its treatment. Almost as soon as behavioural methods were developed, their relevance to treating this clearly defined pattern of behaviour was recognized. The recent literature has charted the evolution of increasingly sophisticated choices of behavioural approach, sometimes in combination with other methods. There has been relatively little work, by comparison, within the family therapy tradition and in other traditions of child therapy. Even so, the overall development of treatment methods may be seen to reflect the shift of focus in models of selective mutism that was described earlier – from intrapsychic processes first to intrafamily issues and then to ways of renegotiating the family's management of its boundary with the outside world. Most recently there have been developments in the use of medication in treatment and in multimodal methods of treatment. We start this part of the book by considering non-behavioural strategies.

Methodological issues

The literature on intervention in selective mutism has a number of defects. Firstly, it does not appear to reflect the full range of work in the area. Most published reports describe treatment successes. There are very few detailed accounts in the literature of the process of failure. Haskell (1964), Brown, Fuller and Gericke (1975) and Rosenberg and Lindblad (1978) are worthy exceptions. Some writers have described the process of failure using one method of intervention before going on to describe success with another method (e.g. Crema and Kerr, 1978; Croghan and Craven, 1982). In general, however, the literature gives little indication that the lessons that can be drawn from failure were learned by those involved, and they are not generally on record.

Secondly, the coverage offered by many writers is partial and inadequate. Some accounts are unclear in the way they describe behaviour before treatment or in their account of the therapeutic intervention itself or in their description of changes in behaviour and adjustment afterwards. Other reports are clear enough but lack detail or precision. For example, Arajarvi (1965) offered a full account of the family background of 12 children treated in an Oslo clinic over a 10-year period and describes significant progress on discharge and follow-up, but did not provide any specific information on the kinds of treatment they had during their hospital stay. Kratochwill (1981), who made this criticism, noted that a similar pattern is found in a number of early reports. In general, later reports of behavioural interventions left fewer major gaps, at least in their accounts of the treatment phase. But some writers still glide over the details of what constitutes an 'improvement' in speaking, e.g. Hill and Scull (1985).

Many accounts have also ignored the later stages of intervention when the focus of the work is on the generalization of improved verbal functioning beyond the first successful setting or people, e.g. Matson et al. (1979). Some authors have expressed the expectation that, once some speech is heard, 'it is just a matter of time until the child's talking generalizes' (Rosenberg and Lindblad, 1978). This is not always the case (see, for example, the account of Sharon aged 7 in Crema and Kerr, 1978). It is important that a detailed account of successful treatment of selective mutism should go on to describe what is done to achieve generalization and maintenance in the everyday situations that the child encounters.

Psychodynamic approaches

Most of the early work on the treatment of selective mutism was informed by a psychodynamic perspective. This tradition has contributed many insights into the phenomenon. At the heart of the classic psychodynamic approach has been the view that the child's problem is not primarily a problem about communication. The restrictions on speaking and communicating are seen as a symptom arising from a severe underlying psychological conflict such as the blocking of a stage of psychosexual development or from inhibitions around the operation of internal object relations. The refusal of speech may mask depression (Hadley, 1994). Words may be experienced by a child as having a symbolic power which makes them dangerous. When words come out of the mouth, they leave an internal space that is not fully in the child's control. To speak is to take a risk, to cut a link that has great emotional significance. For children with unresolved problems of emotional growth the prospect of allowing separation and asserting independence in this way is too intimidating (Rossouw and Lubbe, 1994).

> 'I believe that some of the confusion about this disorder occurs because it is not a single entity: Mutism is a symptom, not a syndrome. It is a compromise formation that occurs when the very act of speaking becomes engaged in conflict. While we may come to learn that biology plays a role in its aetiology, there are always psychodynamic factors that mediate the vicissitudes of the symptom. The child attaches unconscious meaning to the act of speaking. Frequently, speaking becomes 'dangerous' because the child equates it to an act of aggression. Not speaking then becomes the child's way of defending against this forbidden impulse as well as partially expressing it, because silence can also be hostile.'   (Yanof, 1996, p. 80)

Where writers in the behavioural tradition have often concentrated exclusively on the improvement of communication, writers in this tradition have tended to emphasize the range of associated symptoms arising from the hypothesized underlying difficulty. For example, Radford (1977) highlighted a variety of fears behind the belligerent facade put up by Rob (aged 6) – fears of dogs, of stairs, of traffic, of falling down, of being alone. Her perception was that as a toddler he had felt unloved and rejected. He responded angrily to the hostile world by controlling it through the withholding of noise and speech. At the same time he was keeping under control the destructive power of his own aggressive fantasies that he greatly feared. Speech and noise might express his explosive wishes and harm the people on whom he depended for his safety. These intense ambivalent feelings related to an oedipal jealousy and terror of his father and fear of the loss of his mother. Rob was seen for once-weekly psychotherapy for 3 years. The work during this period focused on enabling him to relive and resolve these all-pervasive psychic conflicts in the safety of the transference relationship with the therapist. A particular concern of therapists in this tradition has been that, if the symptom of speech refusal is addressed on its own, other problems may emerge once that one is overcome. Weininger (1987) cited cases in his experience in which mutism was replaced by reading difficulties or psychosomatic complaints or depression. In general, however, symptom substitution of that kind has rarely been reported outside the psychoanalytic literature.

A problem with the psychodynamic approach is that, since the focus of treatment is on issues other than communication, the children's habits of mutism continue. From a behavioural perspective a crucial, and damaging, result is that their status as selective non-speakers continues to be reinforced. In fact, the therapeutic meeting represents a new, dramatic arena for that reinforcement, causing the therapist some frustration (Ruzicka and Sackin, 1974; Shreeve, 1991). For example, the unnamed 7-year-old girl described by Elson et al. (1965) had individual psychotherapy for some months, involving a range of activities, including long walks with the therapist, drawing and clay modelling, and choosing candy and sweets at the candy stand. During all this time she refused to speak to the therapist even once. Many therapists have found that they had to work with such children non-verbally, even teaching them new ways of communicating without speech – a necessary part of the therapeutic strategy if the focus is to be on other issues. The inevitable effect is to reinforce their non-speaking status. As Youngerman (1979) put it, 'By forging other channels of communication, the silence itself is brought into silent question'. Unfortunately the behavioural and social reinforcement of the child's mute stance may outweigh the positive effect Youngerman anticipated. Sometimes, in fact, the child begins to speak to others while maintaining a mute stance with the therapist. It could be that the stimulus control of speech is the key factor in this development (see Chapters 6 and 7).

The use of verbal language is a key mode of communication in psychodynamic therapy and psychoanalysis, in particular to express the therapist's interpretation of the client's speech and behaviour. But it is possible to communicate even interpretations symbolically through other means such as drawing, eye contact, gesture and posture (Greenson, 1961; Blotcky and Looney, 1980) or, with older patients, writing (Subak, West and Carlin, 1982). 'In the end, it is our presence in all its many forms, including our sounds and our words, that opens the way for "more" to happen.' (Woo, 1999, p. 112) Like other workers whose approach will be described later, some psychodynamic therapists and child analysts approach verbal communication with a selectively mute child gradually through non-verbal noises. Yanof (1996) considered that a 'pivotal intervention' in her analytic work with Jeremy (aged 4) was when she began to speak to him in 'another language' as he played in the therapy room:

> I made noises. I made the noises that 4-year-old boys make as they accompany their own play. In fact I wasn't really speaking to Jeremy. More accurately I became the soundtrack to Jeremy's play: a punch landed "POW", a guy fell "THUD", a car collided "CRASH!" – a cacophony of violent sounds. I joined his play; I gave it voice. Within a few days Jeremy began to make noises too – at first tentatively and then more deliberately and with greater abandon. His play had become communicative. It was accompanied by a range of sounds that clearly expressed affect. A man laughed evilly; a woman screamed helplessly; a child voiced surprise; another expressed disgust, all without words. We now had a dialogue about important matters replete with affects. It was as if the spell of the magic mouth had been broken. This is how we "talked" for the next three months when words could not be used. Actually I did not stop talking altogether, but I used my "observing" voice very infrequently. (p. 85)

Psychodynamic approaches are best illustrated through a detailed example. Consider the work of Chethik (1975) with Amy whose treatment began when she was aged 6. At that stage she had been in kindergarten for a year and had not spoken to the teachers or other children once. At home she would whisper occasionally to her parents and siblings but not to anyone else. She was stubborn, passive and uncooperative, plagued by a great number of fears that in some cases led her to extensive superstitious rituals, e.g. when going to bed. Treatment with the male therapist was sustained for 2 years. She did not speak throughout this period but did slowly develop many forms of communication that the author describes as vivid, e.g. drawing, writing, intense play, body gestures, and finally sounds. In the early stages she tended to stick to one corner of the room away from the therapist, playing in a self-absorbed manner with clay. When she moved on to use a doll family, there was a repeated silent routine in which a separation would be followed by a loving reunion. The mother would pick up each child in turn and hug and comfort them. Chethik observed how glad the children seemed to be to get back to their mother and commented how scary it must be to come to his office. At this stage such interpretations were not acknowledged by Amy. She did not even glance in his direction. Throughout the treatment he faced the technical problem that, on the one hand, the patient could not help him hone the accuracy of his interpretations in discussion (he might be 'shooting in the dark') and, on the other hand, she appeared to be awed by his almost magical ability to understand her from her non-verbal material and action fragments.

Slowly Amy began to relax a little in the sessions and to become possessive about her toys in the room. She became fascinated with a pair of scissors and played repeated games in which she put scissors near her mouth and opened and closed both simultaneously. She drew a series of very large pumpkins with prominent mouths and teeth. Chethik interpreted that she was making believe he might be like that – with a big, scary mouth that could bite her. She began to draw dogs with blood spots on them. (She had a long-standing terror of dogs in everyday life.) This was a period when she was reluctant to come to the sessions. Chethik concluded that the fears she had had in the past of the power of her own oral aggression were now being projected onto him: he as the therapist might retaliate by biting. During this period he had also to work with Amy's mother whose ambivalence about the treatment frequently tipped over into covert or open resistance. In the therapy sessions he began to address Amy's fears about oral aggression more directly, discussing the 'Gobble-Gobble feelings' that can make children so scared they will keep their mouths shut very tight. It was then necessary to help her work through unspoken anxieties that talking to others would be a betrayal of her mother.

There were many backward steps as well as advances over the 2-year period of therapy. Without the use of speech it was particularly difficult to do any work on her sexual fantasies and on an early trauma from hospitalization. Her behaviour and drawings alone could not achieve the specificity needed to articulate conflicts in these areas. In spite of progress in some aspects of behaviour and development, she continued to show only a limited capacity for a close and confident relationship with the therapist. On the surface much had improved, but he thought that, although some neurotic aspects of her difficulties had been overcome, she remained psychologically very vulnerable, an individual who might easily revert under stress (e.g. in adolescence) to very primitive ways of relating to others. She still showed omnipotent fantasies in the therapy room. Outside it she was talking quite normally and presenting a fairly well-adjusted persona to the world, but this achievement was seen as fragile in the context of the ambitious and wide-ranging goals of psychodynamic psychotherapy.

Other detailed accounts of psychodynamic treatment of selectively mute children may be found in Mora, De Vault and Schopler (1962), Adams

(1970), Ruzicka and Sackin (1974), Radford (1977), Youngerman (1979), Weininger (1987), Shreeve (1991), Rossouw and Lubbe (1994) and Woo (1999). An account of a full child analysis with a selectively mute patient was published by Yanof (1996). Atoynatan (1986) described an intervention in which dynamic individual psychotherapy was offered to a selectively mute child and her mother separately. Atlas (1993) provided a summary account of psychodynamic therapy in one case in order to illustrate general points that he wished to make about symbol use in selective mutism.

Because there have been fewer such reports in the literature in recent years, reviewers have assumed that this approach to treatment is less commonly adopted now than behavioural and combined approaches (Anstendig, 1998). However, in at least two cities in Switzerland and Germany it was reported in one survey that individual psychotherapy with the child was the single most common form of intervention in three series of cases seen up to 1993 (Steinhausen and Juzi, 1996). This is almost certainly not the case in the UK or North America, but even so 38% of the respondents surveyed by Ford et al. (1998) reported that 'psychotherapy' had been employed in the treatment of selective mutism with their family member. Behavioural and combined approaches may be more common, but psychotherapeutic approaches have not been abandoned.

The psychodynamic perspective has also been employed to inform and guide classroom interventions. For example, Mack and Maslin (1981) reported on work with three selectively mute children in a therapeutic nursery. This establishment was not run wholly on dynamic principles, but it had staff advisers who offered a psychodynamic interpretation of the meaning of the children's play and behaviour. Out of the extensive equipment available each of the three selectively mute children described in this report made considerable use of empty cartons that were sometimes left on the nursery floor or of a cloth tunnel that was big enough to crawl inside. HG (aged 5) would regularly crawl inside the boxes, close the flaps and remain curled up for about 15 minutes. If there were no cartons, he would climb into a very large empty barrel, curling up snugly on its bottom. After a few months he began to vocalize in such venues. 'His sounds were unintelligible, but he persisted in vocalizing whether or not a response was made. Some time after the emergence of this behaviour he had his first intelligible verbal exchange. Having entered an unlit supply closet with an aide, he closed the door and in the dark began to make wordlike sounds.' He repeated this behaviour and generalized it to the classroom itself. Soon afterwards he began to use words in talking to one of the classroom aides, and then slowly in conversation with most other staff, always speaking in a low voice using short phrases. He continued to play in the boxes and would still make unintelligible sounds while inside them.

The authors offered a psychodynamic explanation of this behaviour. They suggested that a 'claustral experience' in the classroom may help a child towards open communication for two reasons:

- If mute behaviour constitutes a withdrawal from a world seen as hostile or dangerous (Adams and Glasner, 1954), the enclosure offers a protective barrier within which the child is free to experiment with speech safely.
- The use of boxes may be relevant where children withhold speech because they are fearful of the destructive power of their own aggressive urges that might be released or expressed through speaking and might lead to consequences they cannot control. In this case it is hypothesized that the carton or closet or tunnel may provide safe containment for the child's aggressive urges. (An alternative social behavioural explanation would emphasize that the opportunity to avoid making eye contact while speaking could have facilitated speech in this situation.)

Another application of the psychodynamic perspective to classroom management may be found in Gemelli (1983).

Play therapy

There are very few published reports of the use of play therapy outside the psychodynamic tradition as an intervention strategy in the treatment of selective mutism. Bozigar and Hansen (1984) established a small therapy group for four selectively mute girls aged 6–9 years. 'The plan was to help the children examine their mutism in school in a therapeutic setting where they would be free to understand their anxieties, inhibitions and the consequences of their behaviour' (p. 479). Although the work included clay modelling and the use of play materials such as dolls, jump ropes and board games, a key element in its success was planned desensitization within a behavioural framework, so their intervention is covered in the next chapter.

In the view of Barlow, Strother and Landreth (1986) it was crucial to their work with Amy, a 5-year-old girl with selective mutism, that group therapy could 'provide an atmosphere in which the child feels safe and where there is no pressure to talk' (p. 50). In addition, they drew on insights from family therapy in planning sibling group therapy. They observed that Amy did not need to take responsibility for herself because her older brother, Ben, aged 9, 'was the responsible one . . . talked and played for both of them' (p. 47). A key element in their work with her consisted of helping Amy to become more confident and independent and to share control of play sessions and the play area.

Roe (1993) faced a greater challenge in creating the separate, 'safe' environment required for group play therapy, as it took place in a spare classroom in the nursery/infant school where she was working as a language support teacher. 'The role I adopted was that of a "senior" group member, not that of teacher. I sat on the carpet with the children, to be at their level. I participated in activities with them and built on ideas initiated by them, as well as initiating activities myself.' In this way she hoped to 'establish a relaxed environment in which all means of communicating - verbal and non-verbal – were accepted and encouraged' (p. 134). The sessions were short (20 minutes) and were held two to three times a week. Brief games played in pairs or as a whole group were planned in such a way that the children developed awareness of and confidence in their own bodies, together with trust in relating to others in a protected environment, and gradually moved from non-verbal to verbal communication. The children, about half of whom had English as an additional language, included individuals who were shy and withdrawn as well as some who were selectively mute. Roe ascribed their good progress partly to being identified early before the problems of communication in school were 'too firmly set'. She suggested, in addition, that the group setting provided an opportunity for the children to break out of a self-image as 'quiet' or 'mute'. They can 'in an environment of acceptance, begin to explore different ways of being and relating . . . they can experience new aspects of themselves and decide if they want to incorporate these into their self-image' (p. 139). (Similar points were made by Stephenson (1993), who described the use of drama in group work with children and adolescents.)

It will be evident that, for different reasons, it was important for each of those authors that they were working with the children in a group rather than on an individual basis. Cook (1997) argued a strong case for the value of individual work in this context. She explained the advantages of using play therapy for selective mutism by reference to the specific curative powers of play proposed by Schaefer (1993). He suggested that the therapeutic benefits of play therapy derive from fourteen factors of which she focuses on four in her account of key therapeutic effects in work with children who are selectively mute:

- communication for the expansion of a child's verbal and non-verbal repertoire
- overcoming resistance against the development of a collaborative alliance
- competency for experience of mastery in play and communicative experiences with a consequent growth in self-esteem
- 'positive emotion' to enable expression of a full range of emotions in social interaction including adaptive management of anxiety.

Cook's approach can be illustrated through her analysis of what is seen by many as the Achilles heel of individual therapy with selectively mute children – verbal communication. She acknowledged that an insistence on straightforward verbal expression might lead to the sessions revolving around the child's response set of mutism and withdrawal but continued:

Fortunately, play therapy views the expression of the child in play as a full expression of the self in childhood. Play is as valuable as verbal expression for communication and even more so in assessing and intervening in the emotional realm . . . As children play out emotions they can become aware, through the therapist's interactions and reflections, of the emotional content associated with their restrictions in affect, behaviour, and speech. The opportunity to express a wider range of affects and behaviours evolves as they determine control of their varied emotional levels and become less constricted in their behaviour. This allows increased self-awareness and development of a range of degrees of self-control and self-expression . . . There is no need to await verbal communication, for the child and therapist are in constant ongoing communication through the play. The level of communication may remain within the play metaphor or be drawn to the level of the child's involvement and personal content. Careful bridging is required, however, to avoid confrontational material that could hinder the communicative growth. The level of overt and direct communication from the child may initially be subtle or may be responded to as if intended and be rewarded with more consistent responsiveness. Movement, postures, and gestures provide entrée for responsive communication through mirroring the pace and level at which the child initiates communication as well as providing alternatives in expression for the child to emulate. Offering the child too much verbiage or too quick a pace can result in a break in the rhythm to which the child has become accustomed and comfortable. The pace and responsiveness will vary from child to child and can be viewed in comparison to their historical patterns of speech, fully expressed possibly only at home, and never expressed in other social environments. The initial vocalizations of the child may evolve through a variety of means such as noisemaking, repetitive sounds, humming, whispers, or verbalizations ranging from monosyllables or phrases to complete thoughts. However, as this phenomenon emerges it becomes only one part of the communicative content incorporated in the ongoing total communication of playing out oneself in the here and now. Over time, the full pattern of communication becomes an envelope within which the child and therapist are increasingly mutually involved in synchrony. The ongoing play also continues to provide content that may be communicated jointly by action and reaction, emotion and emotional response, and comment and reply. The integration of play, thought, emotion, and expression encourages evolution of a more fully experiencing and expressive child characterized by active involvement and open communication. (pp. 94–95)

Cook saw the value of combined approaches and made clear that ideas from behavioural and family therapy had influenced her thinking. But she asserted that the success of her work in nine cases derived from the fact that she 'utilized centrally and foremost individual client-centred child play therapy with an adjunct parent and teacher consultation model' (p. 100). Once children could communicate easily with the now-familiar adult therapist, careful attention was paid to generalization of their new confidence to communication with 'unfamiliar adults and with peers in a variety of forms and in age-expected situations'. We can note that stimulus fading played a part in some cases as 'providing a direct communicative transition through other dyads or through groups' (p. 95). But the flavour of what Cook felt to be the core of the approach is caught more faithfully by the use of metaphor in this quotation from one of the children: 'There was a fish who always swam under the water. He learned how to swim to the top and peep out and then to leap out and look around and now he is a flying fish.' (p. 100)

Art therapy

Since non-verbal means of communication and expression have been so crucial in psychodynamic psychotherapy with children who are selectively mute, it might be expected that art therapy and music therapy could have much to offer. The literature is sparse. In music therapy the only published paper concerns work with an adult woman who was selectively mute (Aigen, 1990). But, in the case of art therapy at least, the limited published literature does suggest some interesting and worthwhile issues for future exploration. Of course, elements of art therapy often feature as a supplement to verbal psychotherapy with selectively mute patients. Examples include Heuyer and Morgenstern (1927) (cited in Landgarten, 1975), Mora, De Vault and Schopler, (1962) and Chethik (1975) whose work was described earlier in this chapter. Art therapy as the primary mode of therapy is less commonly reported.

In art therapy visual images play a central part. Writers vary in how they interpret the process of creating them. Some have seen artistic activity in the therapeutic setting primarily as a 'therapeutic occupation', a relaxing diversion or distraction from disturbing thoughts. Others (latterly the dominant group in British art therapy) have emphasized the role of image-making as a means of communicating innermost feelings. The therapeutic setting comprises three elements – the patient, the therapist and the art work. In this context there will be strong feelings of transference and countertransference, as in any psychotherapeutic relationship, but there will also be a focus on the visual objects that are created as that relationship develops. That focus is thought to enable the art therapist to help in situations where traditional 'insight-providing' methods are inadequate (Waller, 1991, Chapters 1 and 26). Its potential value for work with selectively mute children may be seen in a general statement of faith by one of the profession's pioneers, Irene Champernown:

> More than 25 years ago I became acutely aware of the fact that words, particularly in prose, were an extremely difficult medium through which to convey our deepest experiences of life. It was clear that the mind was filled with visual, aural and bodily images which were suitable containers for emotions and ideas that were otherwise inexpressible. The experience of these images was not only a means of communication between one human being and another, though that is something we experience here most

strongly, but it is also a way of communication from the unconscious levels
of experience to a more conscious understanding in the individual himself.
(Champernown, 1963, quoted in Waller, 1991)

The potential of this approach to therapy for work with selective
mutism will be illustrated through two examples.

In an unconventional paper, Hesse (1981) concentrated on the formal
analysis of drawings in the case of a 4-year-old girl who did not speak at all.
He argued that visual media could offer more than an additional channel
(besides language) for absorbing and expressing the emotional burden a
child is carrying. These media can also promote 'graphical conceptualization', which will facilitate more adequate verbal intercourse. This claim
assumes that children who are mute have particular problems of conceptualization. There is no evidence for that in selective mutism. It is relevant
that the girl in Hesse's report may have been generally rather than selectively mute. However, his account of the therapeutic intervention offers
ideas that seem relevant to selective mutism. He analysed the formal features of the child's drawings, such as the composition of her work and her
use of the surface space, form and colour. Thematic and figurative content
were ignored in the analysis (and were in any case sparse). Hesse identified two co-existing main styles, both described as 'non-communicative'.
One style was emotionally restrained, expressing defensive introversion,
and the other was emotionally unrestrained, expressing aggressive extra-
version. Her drawings, like her behaviour, appeared to show a reactive
withdrawal from situations in which she could only make an aggressive
response. Perhaps she feared to do so, sensing lack of control. The ultimate aim of the intervention was to help the child develop graphic
concepts related to visual reality and then convert these into verbal concepts. Use would be made of the potential that any drawing activity has to
encourage the structuring and emotional control of an aspect of external
reality. Hesse aimed to channel the aggression shown in one style and
loosen the inhibiting use of enclosure in the other style.

The girl was encouraged to work without others present and standing
rather than sitting, so that she could move freely in front of a large verti-
cal surface. Liquid poster colours and big brushes were put at her
disposal, replacing the rigid crayons she had been using before. An assistant whom she appeared to like stood by her as she worked, with a brief
not to ask questions or solicit speech. She did not comment except for
teaching a vocabulary for colour, shape, etc.

> Some anticipated effects could . . . be observed. The vertical position caused
> the liquid colours to spill and 'burst through' the former rigidly defined
> shapes. In order to avoid frustration these 'walls' were to be re-established
> with the cautious support of the assistant. This cooperation somehow less-
> ened their self-defensive character and helped loosen the self-imposed
> strictness. The corporal gratification of freely splashing and daubing colours
> replaced the stabbing violence encountered before. While seemingly of a

purely regressive nature, this activity was also intended to permit a fresh start at the preverbal stage and to gradually develop speech by integration of emotional expression and verbal communication.

(Hesse, 1981, p. 181)

After two months of work along these lines her drawings showed significant changes and a new style emerged – more flexible and continuous in execution, more rhythmical in composition, using the borders of a space more effectively, and varying the choice of colour according to the subject. Within another month she was speaking fluently and 'was able to communicate with others by word, touch and regard. Today she attends a regular school.' Hesse does not claim that his intervention was the only factor in these changes. Much of the improvement is attributed to the therapeutic activities and surroundings of the special education kindergarten where the work took place. but the diagnosis and prognosis formulated on the basis of a formal analysis of her art work were largely confirmed.

A contrasting approach closer to the mainstream of art therapy tradition was employed by Landgarten (1975) with an older child, Cora (aged 7). She offered a wider range of activities (including drawing, painting, storytelling and collage) and placed an explicit focus on the content as well as the form of the child's productions. The use of collage enabled Cora to introduce quite complex themes. She would then tell a story about her selected pictures (e.g. focusing on adults' thoughts of sexual infidelity). An interesting feature of this work was that Cora was initially seen together with one or two of her older siblings (she was the fourth of a family of six). This was intended to make the treatment less threatening. It also provided an arena for working through problems of family secrecy and intimacy. (The issue of child protection is not explicitly discussed.) At first Cora could neither portray members of her family together nor work collaboratively with them on a task. She could only draw and tell stories about individual little girls on their own in the picture. Sometimes she seemed to use these stories for more than expressing her own fantasies and feelings. 'They served as a creative trial for something that Cora would later attempt outside therapy.' One example was playing with other children in their houses rather than her own.

Landgarten suggests that with this child art was not used so much for interpretation as a means of self-expression and as a springboard for verbal communication. It was combined with behavioural strategies of a kind to be described in the next two chapters for managing her step-by-step approach to bolder efforts at talking to a wider group of people. In the first instance, however, the sessions of individual and joint art therapy were seen as 'providing a medium that was less direct and therefore less frightening than speech'. Her collages and drawings helped her towards being able to use words for direct communication with other people. (For another example of art therapy as the primary mode of treatment for a selectively mute child see Howard, 1963.)

Family therapy

Because selective mutism tends to develop in families that show unusual patterns of interaction, it seems reasonable to expect that family work will have a contribution to make to treatment. It might even be hoped that family therapy could tackle the roots of the problem. The assumptions about causality behind this view are implicit in some psychodynamic analyses, even where there is no account of a whole-family intervention as such (e.g. Meijer, 1979). It is striking that, in fact, very little work on selective mutism has been conducted within the main family therapy traditions. There is general acknowledgement that, whatever approach is adopted, some family involvement is essential, but often this has simply meant an adaptation of traditional, individually focused methods (e.g. Pustrom and Speers, 1964). In fact, some of those who have advocated family therapy approaches appear to have held a relatively unsophisticated notion of what family work might entail. For example, Goll, who introduced the influential concept of the role of the 'ghetto family' into discussions of selective mutism, devoted only a very short section of his key paper to treatment strategies and offered simplistic guidelines for family work that do not address the complex and subtle systemic issues revealed in his earlier analysis (Goll, 1979, pp. 67–68). A fully developed family therapy perspective must involve a rethinking not only of the development of the behaviour but also of how it is described to members of the family and how they are invited to take part in therapy. (For an example of workers who could appreciate this perspective but chose – or were compelled – to work differently, see Crema and Kerr, 1978.)

Some workers have argued that neither family therapy nor individual therapy is efficient on its own. They believe that treatment methods must be combined to achieve effective change and that it is necessary to bring about changes in the family system if any changes achieved in the child's speaking habits through behaviour modification or individual therapy are to be maintained (Rosenberg and Lindblad, 1978). There is no firm research evidence to back these assertions, but there is an interesting analogy in this argument with the model of school phobia proposed by Blagg (1987). It could be claimed that individual work tackles the 'precipitating factors' of selective mutism and family work tackles the 'maintaining factors' (see Chapter 3). As Rosenberg and Lindblad express it, 'The importance of the family approach is to help modify family patterns and structures so that whatever led to the development of the problem in the child is changed, thereby permitting the positive change in the child to continue to unfold.'

A number of family therapists working with selective mutism agree with Rosenberg and Lindblad that the most effective approach is to combine family work with a behavioural intervention focused on the child's talking to others. (Rare exceptions are Meyers (1984) and Tatem and

Delcampo (1995) who employed individual play therapy alongside family sessions.) The family work is typically directed first towards tackling
the problems of an enmeshed relationship between the child and a parent (usually the mother), the isolation or marginalization of a family
member (often the father), blocking of open expression of feelings, or
general over-protectiveness. For example, Afnan and Carr (1989) worked
very slowly to detach Mrs C. from her over-involvement with her daughter Jenny (aged 6). With the participation of both parents they devised a
treatment strategy for her mutism. The plan led Mrs C. to reduce the
time she spent as a voluntary aide in Jenny's classroom. At the same time
it gave Mr C. a central role in implementing a planned star chart reinforcement programme at home each evening. The insights that lay
behind this allocation of roles came from family therapy, but the changes
were introduced in the service of an explicit behavioural programme. In
effect, the behavioural programme itself fulfilled the function of a
between-sessions task in family therapy. (This programme is described in
more detail in Chapter 6.)

It has been commented that proponents of family therapy often focus
only on the family system when seeking to identify disposing and maintaining factors in selective mutism and when planning treatment. The
family as a whole becomes the 'client' and is put under pressure to
change. It is possible to adopt a different perspective. The child's
mutism is seen to make parents, who are already very anxious people,
even more anxious. They feel failures as parents and are embarrassed by
their child's behaviour. Involving them as 'facilitators' in a behavioural
programme rather than as 'clients' needing therapy is a different
approach to work with the family which emphasizes their ability to
understand their children's needs and their competence to help them.
Re-reading Afnan and Carr's account of their work with Jenny's family
from that perspective places more emphasis on the active and specific
roles that each parent adopted in the work with Jenny and less emphasis on the therapists' attempts to influence family dynamics by their
ascription of these roles.

Often, of course, the work on family systems and family myths focuses
not on the individual behavioural programme but on interactions during
the family's meetings with the therapist. For example, Rosenberg and
Lindblad (1978) achieved a breakthrough with Tony (aged 6) when his
father manoeuvred his way downstairs in spite of being 'sick' in bed and
in spite of his wife's covert attempts to exclude him. Lindblad-Goldberg
(1986), working with Jerry (aged 5), employed a board game in four
sequential family sessions ostensibly to facilitate speech from Jerry but
effectively 'to help the parents (mother and new stepfather) support each
other, express conflict, and resolve differences, always with the stated goal
of helping Jerry'. Roberts (1984) used a highly formalized ritual to mark
the end of treatment for Sara (aged 14). The family buried in the hospital

grounds a secure box with a video clip of how Sara used to be (unable to walk on her own as well as mute) and written descriptions of how her parents used to help her walk. The past was buried but in a way that made it accessible if it were ever needed. This ritual helped to complete the total replacement of the old family myth that Sara was totally helpless and needed her mother's selfless care in order to function.

In a contrasting approach drawing from other practices within the family therapy tradition, Hoffman and Laub (1986) suggested that too much attention had often been given to the children's anxiety and family dynamics and too little attention paid to the controlling, manipulating, negativistic passive-aggressive aspect of their behaviour. They involved Lily (aged 4), her elder brother Eli, their parents and grandparents in a series of family meetings and challenges, relying heavily on paradoxical interventions. Their strategy exploited the potential of having two co-therapists present, making the female therapist a 'good' person for the family (sympathetic towards Lily and positive about her ability to change) and the male therapist a 'bad' person (disparaging of Lily's immaturity and pessimistic about her future). After some initial exploratory meetings the 'bad' therapist bet first with his co-therapist and then Eli that Lily would fail to meet a series of challenges in a simple hierarchy of increasingly demanding situations. The siblings (and their parents) took great delight in his losing the bets.

Hoffman and Laub conceived of Lily's mutism as a source of power and control for her within the family. The provocation of the 'bad' therapist upset the balance so that she needed to re-establish control. By winning the bet for the family she achieved this 'but in a more constructive and appropriate way'. The support of the 'good' therapist reduced her anxiety and strengthened her self-confidence and self-esteem so that she was able to meet the challenge. Within the family, of course, all members had been provoked to unite in allowing her a new role. The threat of the 'bad' therapist's poor opinion was greater than the threat of a change in the family's internal balance.

'Paradoxical' techniques may only be justified in the context of a particular view of family dynamics. As a family doctor Furst (1989) adopted a rather different game-based approach to disturbing, long-standing family patterns of interaction. He gave his highly competitive 10-year-old patient the opportunity to beat him at a card game which she passionately enjoyed. But she could not defeat him until she had explained some of the rules to him. His family were complicit in that they did not speak for her. She soon followed her first words, 'You have to pick up three cards from the card bank', by generalizing speech to other situations.

Overall family therapists have contributed to work with selective mutism rich insights and strategies that appear to have great potential value beyond their own area of practice. It will be useful to bear these in mind when considering the approaches examined in the next two chapters.

Residential treatment

Residential treatment involves a major intervention in the life of the child and the family. Often children are away from home for extended periods. Hospital stays may last many months, in extreme cases a year and a half (Roberts, 1984), or even 3 years (Wassing, 1973). Stays in residential school will typically last much longer. The outcome of residential treatment has been variable. In a notable review of a series of cases in Oslo, Wergeland (1979) found that the children whose parents refused residential treatment did better than those who had it. Some case studies report little change in the overall situation after discharge (e.g. Subak, West and Carlin, 1982). In some individual cases, however, significant improvements have been achieved (e.g. Wassing (1973), Munford et al. (1976) and Roberts (1984) working with young people in their teens and Elson et al. (1965), Matson et al. (1979) and Maskey (2001) working with younger children). These cases almost all date back many years, as this form of treatment is not generally favoured today. One problem with the reports on older children is that they often fail to make clear what treatment had been attempted before the child was admitted to a residential facility.

Some of the children and young people who have been hospitalized or sent to boarding special school were clearly at a point of crisis before admission. It was not possible for them to remain at home and receive effective treatment. For example, Sara (aged 14) was not only selectively mute but had refused to walk by herself for 2 years. Her parents would crouch behind her to move her legs physically in order that she could be mobile (Roberts, 1984). Owen (aged 14) had been mute for 10 years when he was admitted to hospital. Three earlier attempts at intervention had failed. His parents requested admission with the complaint that he refused to change his clothes, often locked himself in their only bathroom for 45 minutes at a time, and still refused to speak outside the home (Youngerman, 1979). In such cases there is a defensible case for treatment away from the home setting. However, some of the reports in the literature describe a speedy move into hospital or residential placement after what seems to have been a cursory attempt at home-based treatment. Of course, treatment for a child while living at home requires the cooperation of the child's family, and there are many reasons why the parents of children with selective mutism may resist treatment and many ways that they can sabotage it even if not openly refusing it. But, reading the early literature, it is hard to avoid the conclusion that some professionals allowed their frustration over initial treatment failure to lead them surprisingly quickly into an excessively intrusive and disruptive form of intervention. This is not so evident in the more recent literature.

In some cases it is not obvious that hospitalization was an important feature of the treatment at all: the ward appears simply to have provided a location from which conventional outpatient treatment could be arranged easily. What, in fact, are the key features of residential placement when it is successful and necessary in work with selectively mute children? The first important feature is the removal of the child from the family environment where the contingencies maintaining a mute pattern of behaviour are strongly entrenched. The second important feature is the total control that the therapists temporarily have over the child's environment. This offers them possibilities that are not open to others – for example, control over a range of major reinforcements such as avoiding a noxious stimulus on a daily basis (Shaw, 1971) or (more positively) allowing a child to go home for a weekend (Crema and Kerr, 1978) or Christmas (Roberts, 1984). A third important feature is the opportunity to facilitate social interaction with trained staff and peers throughout the day during leisure and mealtimes as well as in school. Carradice (1988) conveys the potential impact of these opportunities in an anecdote of Roger (aged 16) at a residential assessment centre. Roger was completely mute on admission and never spoke to adults there – except that towards the end he would mutter a comment, often a swear word, when a member of staff came into a room. He would then quickly leave amid peals of laughter from other boys.

> Late one night, when I was going off duty, I discovered what had happened. Passing his dormitory, I heard the sound of voices – Roger was talking to the other lads; not just the odd word or phrase but whole sentences, as clearly and effectively as anybody else. Every night, apparently, the boys had been talking to and with him, slowly pulling the thoughts and words out of his reluctant head. At their urging he had been dropping us the odd comment, a great game which everyone had thoroughly enjoyed.

These features (separation from home, total control of the environment, and a new social setting) each played an important part in the rehabilitation of the most damaged young people in this literature (e.g. Kevin described by Hayden, 1983 and Sara described by Roberts, 1984). At the same time the risks of residential placement are great. The parents are (temporarily) supplanted. The child's release from family pressures may facilitate some kinds of personal change at the expense of leaving the family problem untouched. It may then be very difficult to maintain any individual change that the child has achieved after a return home. For this reason Roberts (1984) combined family therapy with inpatient treatment and worked hard to prevent a divergence of effort or a breakdown of communication between the two. It was not easy. Members of the family felt hurt when Sara talked first to 'strangers' in the psychiatric unit rather than to one of them. Roberts and her colleagues sought to bridge the gap in various ways, paying careful attention to both practical and symbolic issues and facilitating future communication. For example, Sara was very interested in animals, and they persuaded her parents to buy a pet parakeet that they would keep at home. In the unit Sara privately made tape recordings for the bird, saying the same word over and over again for the bird to repeat. The tapes were taken home after family visits to the ward, and the parents played them for the bird. When Sara went home on a visit, she spent some time alone with the bird, coaching it. Eventually she was making tapes not just for the bird but for family members, then speaking to them face-to-face. Initially the most striking feature of this part of Roberts' treatment plan appears to be the imaginative use of the pet. Sadly, however, an even more striking feature is that the mundane planning of family–hospital contact and family visits is rarely described in this literature. Treatment plans that are otherwise very careful and detailed, such as those of Wassing (1973), Matson et al. (1979) and Cunningham et al. (1983), simply omit this dimension.

In some cases further problems arise over planning for the child's return home from hospital or boarding school. If there is no provision there for changing the contingencies that reinforced mutism previously, the pattern may quickly be re-established. This was the case, for example, when Nicola (aged 12), who was described by Maskey (2001), returned to a school that could not cater for her learning difficulties. The hospital team had determined that her cognitive and educational performance was well below what would be expected at her age, but her parents and some of her teachers were reluctant to accept a change of school regime as they put her problems with the curriculum down to her previous failure to speak. Her progress in hospital had been uneven, but such as it was, it was lost when she returned to the same school situation as before.

Conclusions

Therapists from outside the behavioural tradition have frequently found selective mutism very difficult to treat, and in recent years behavioural methods have been strongly favoured. But this review has shown that much can be achieved and much has been learned employing non-behavioural methods. Those working in the psychodynamic tradition have given eloquent testimony to the importance of the other symptoms associated with selectively mute behaviour and to the intensity of adults' negative reactions to children who will not talk to them. It was not surprising to find that success could be achieved through the medium of art therapy in which visual images play a central part rather than verbal interaction. For some children this provides a medium that is less direct and so less frightening than speech – a step towards using words for direct communication with other people.

Work in family therapy has underlined the importance of taking account of family dynamics when planning any form of intervention and has suggested some effective ways of doing so. The review has indicated that residential treatment will only have a role in the treatment of selective mutism in extreme circumstances and has indicated particular issues to which those involved in residential treatment need to give special attention, e.g. home–centre links.

All of the insights from non-behavioural perspectives (and the strategies associated with them) are underplayed or lost altogether in many accounts of behavioural approaches. This will be evident from the review of the development of behavioural methods in Chapter 6. Examples of how such issues can be addressed within a behavioural framework will be given in Chapters 7 and 8. For example, the strategy proposed in Chapter 7 is likely to bring about changes not only in stimulus control of a child's habits of speaking to others but also in their family's way of interacting with the outside world (especially schools) – and perhaps changes in their teachers' way of interacting with the parents.

Chapter 6
The development of behavioural approaches: a historical review

This chapter traces a dramatic increase over a period of four decades in the use of behavioural approaches to help selectively mute children. To some extent this reflected the general growth in the use of behaviour therapy from the mid-1950s, but there were also specific factors relating to selective mutism. There have always been attempts by parents and teachers to change children's behaviour and patterns of speech through punishment or reward. Occasionally behavioural techniques have been used by psychodynamic therapists, although they run counter to the therapists' views on the causes of the children's mute behaviour. But it was not until the mid-1960s that the first attempts were made to apply theoretical models of learning to helping selectively mute children. The initial work appeared in the literature in a small number of experimental reports and a larger number of anecdotal case studies. These early reports are repeatedly cited in later studies.

In the second period, starting from around 1971, there was a heightened interest in reporting successful outcomes. The number of published reports increased, using for the most part operant behaviour models. As confidence in the effectiveness of behavioural approaches grew, concern began to be expressed about methodological and ethical issues. Subsequent work met most of the earlier criticisms of poor methodology, although the outcome measures that were used were often inadequate.

Different learning theories and models of learning have been applied, sometimes in an eclectic way. Earlier work often tried to link beliefs about the causes of the behaviour with the selection of a particular form of intervention. Later there was a greater focus on operant models with increased emphasis on using assessment of behaviour as the basis for intervention, and, through improved methodology, establishing an empirical research base. However, there have also been reports combining behavioural intervention and family therapy or the use of medication and studies which draw on social learning theory and cognitive behaviour therapy. The purpose of this chapter is to give the background to the development of behavioural approaches and to outline some of the more important methodological issues.

Behavioural approaches

The basis of behavioural approaches

The term 'behavioural approaches' is used here to encompass a wide variety of methods described variously as 'behaviour therapy', 'applied behaviour analysis' and 'behaviour modification', terms which are often used interchangeably (Calhoun and Turner, 1981). Kazdin (1978) offered a statement of the features they share that remains useful today:

- There will be a focus on the present factors which determine behaviour and on the relationship between target behaviours and the environment in which they occur.
- The effectiveness of the intervention will be evaluated through observations of changes in behaviour. Measurement will be repeated or continuous (in contrast to the strategy of one-off pretreatment and post-treatment assessment associated with some other approaches to treatment).
- The aim of the intervention will be to provide opportunities for the child to learn adaptive behaviour in place of previously learned maladaptive behaviours.
- The intervention will be 'tailor made' to the individual through careful assessment which is specific in its description and through measurement of the target behaviours. It is intended that assessment and intervention will be much more tightly related than diagnosis and treatment are in psychodynamic approaches.
- The intervention will be described in operational terms, with specific description of treatments and measures so that it can be replicated by another worker.
- There will be clear links to learning theory and experimental psychology as a source of ideas about techniques and experimental design.

Work on different ways of learning suggested different behavioural approaches. For example, classical conditioning highlights the association between a stimulus and a response, as in the well-known example of the eyeblink response. The reflex action, blinking, can become conditioned to a new stimulus. Normally people blink if there is a sudden puff of air directed at their eyes, but do not blink if a light suddenly grows brighter. However, if air is puffed into the eye just before a light gets brighter, the blinking response (previously an unconditioned response) becomes conditioned to the increase in brightness (the conditioned stimulus) and becomes a conditioned response. When this is applied to selective mutism, it is usually envisaged that an association has developed between speaking to strangers and feeling anxious. In behavioural work with children who are selectively mute the classical conditioning paradigm has been a point of reference for therapists using explanatory terms like anxiety, avoidance and phobia. In general this group of therapists have tried to link intervention to the causes of the behaviour. They have employed therapeutic techniques such as counterconditioning which consists of pairing a pleasant experience with a carefully sequenced introduction of, say, an object that is feared. The sequence is arranged to ensure that the exposure to the fearful situation is gradually increased while a positive emotional 'set' is maintained. The aim is to reduce the effects of the feared object and to reverse the original conditioning of the fear response. For example, to countercondition a child's fear of all white furry objects we could put him at a table with his favourite food. As he eats, we would bring in a white furry toy, first at a distance, and move it closer to him gradually (cf. Jones (1924), quoted by Gelfand, 1979).

Systematic desensitization is a form of counterconditioning which uses a hierarchy of situations that have an increasing effect in inducing fear. In this approach the aim is to elicit a response incompatible with anxiety in the presence of the fear-arousing stimulus (Wolpe, 1958). For example, a person who is afraid of spiders would gradually be helped to experience feelings incompatible with feeling anxious. The incompatible response most frequently trained is relaxation. Patients would be asked to imagine a hierarchy of increasingly fearsome spider situations, perhaps culminating in the actual presence of spiders. When they can handle spiders without anxiety, the fear response has been extinguished. As will be seen later, forms of systematic desensitization have been used in the treatment of selective mutism.

When that approach is used in this context, the therapist must take account of the fact that selectively mute children are not 'willing' patients like the adults seeking treatment for spider phobia. Selectively mute children have found their own ways of reducing anxiety by avoiding speech. For this reason, when desensitization is used alone in the treatment of selective mutism, it is necessarily an extended and very gradual process. (See the example of Scott's work with Linda described in Chapter 7.)

The operant model of behaviour has been the other major paradigm influencing the development of behavioural approaches. According to that model, the probability of behaviour occurring again depends on its past and present consequences and also its past and present antecedents. It is common to employ a framework in which three elements are analysed – antecedents, behaviour and consequences (ABC). If that framework is applied to selective mutism, the antecedents are the stimuli which act as cues for speaking and not speaking, and the consequences are those experiences that strengthen or weaken the relationship between the stimuli and speech. 'Stimulus control' of speech depends on reinforcing speaking and not speaking differentially in the presence of certain stimuli. For example, a young child who has a stomach ache may reply readily to her mother about it in the presence of her baby brother at home but not in the presence of an unfamiliar doctor in his surgery. The key stimuli can include both people and settings. Changing stimulus control may involve introducing new stimuli so gradually that they can barely be discriminated from the stimuli which facilitate speaking. Reinforcing the verbal behaviour which occurs in association with both the old and the new stimuli will strengthen the relationship. Gradually the old stimuli can be faded out while the behaviour is maintained. Stimulus fading has proved to be an important concept in work on selective mutism.

An example of stimulus fading from a different area of psychology is given in the account by Wickings et al. (1974) of a boy with learning difficulties who would only drink from a spoon and never from a cup. The stimulus control of drinking had to be shifted from spoon to cup. Over a period of several weeks the shape of the spoon was deepened and the handle was first shortened and then bent over to become the handle of the spoon/cup while the boy continued to drink from the gradually changing 'spoon'. Because of the need to make the spoon/cups this process took several months. Care was taken to ensure that drinking from a cup was generalized to other settings. Follow-up after 6 months and again after 4 years showed the new behaviour was maintained. The crucial aspect of stimulus fading appears to be the fact that the change in stimulus control is made very gradually while reinforcement continues.

Behaviour is of course strengthened by both positive and negative reinforcement, as shown in Table 6.1.

Table 6.1 Application of positive and negative reinforcement

	Pleasant consequences	Unpleasant consequences
Apply	Increase behaviour (positive reinforcement)	Decrease behaviour (punishment)
Remove	Decrease behaviour	Increase behaviour (negative reinforcement)

Application of positive and negative reinforcement

In reports on selective mutism there are very frequent references to eliciting speech through positive reinforcement. At the same time it is important to remember that not speaking is also strongly influenced by positive reinforcement. In many target situations, such as school, selectively mute children receive an immense amount of positive reinforcement for not speaking, both when they receive extra attention during attempts to make them speak and when their non-verbal communication inevitably elicits a response from others. When, on the other hand, attempts are made to ignore their mutism and their non-verbal communication, these will often be inconsistent. The result is that there is intermittent positive reinforcement for staying mute – a pattern of reinforcement that is known to strengthen behaviour and make it particularly resistant to change. At the same time the children may experience considerable anxiety about speaking outside the home. Then remaining silent, even under great pressure to talk, relieves that anxiety and negatively reinforces non-speaking by removing an unpleasant consequence associated with speaking. Again the likelihood of the mute behaviour recurring is increased.

Influence of social learning theory

During the late 1970s and 1980s an increasingly influential paradigm in work on selective mutism, as in other fields, was social learning theory (Bandura, 1969, 1977). This approach embodies elements of both classical conditioning and operant learning. Initially it too emphasized the importance of direct experience of antecedents and consequences in learning behaviour. Where it differs is in the important role given to central cognitive processes which mediate the links between external stimuli and behaviour. It is envisaged that learning can take place solely through cognitive activities and that behaviour can be controlled through thoughts and speech. Almost all behaviour that is learned through direct experience can also be learned through observation by processes such as imitation, modelling and identification. This has clear relevance to the environmental influences, especially of maternal behaviour, in the families of selectively mute children. Imitation and modelling of family members and identification with them may be important in initially establishing and then maintaining selective mutism.

Modelling was found to be more effective than providing reassuring information or physical contact in the control of fear of snakes (Blanchard 1970). It has been used in the treatment of children's fears, often through observation of live or filmed peer models coping well in the feared situations. It appears to be most effective in helping children with fears when they can identify with the children who model the desired behaviour, because they show that they share the fears but manage to overcome them. Peer modelling of appropriate verbal behaviour is of course available to children who are selectively mute in their everyday lives, but it has no effect. It is assumed that this is because the other children are perceived by the mute children as different from them. Probably family members act as the most influential models for social interactions for them, rather than their peers. Whatever the reason, the practical effect is the same: peer modelling has a very weak effect on their behaviour. It cannot be the crux of behavioural intervention as it has been with some other childhood problems, such as specific fears.

Cognitive-behavioural approaches

As noted in Chapter 4, another form of modelling, self-modelling, appears to be an effective technique with some selectively mute children. This technique extends social learning theory to include elements of cognitive behaviour therapy. Cognitive behaviour theorists had emphasized the part played by images, thoughts and self-verbalization in developing and maintaining phobic and other maladaptive behaviour. Understanding of cognitive disturbances in anxious children has developed rapidly over the last 10–15 years. Biased attention and memory processes, negative thinking and worrying are some of the factors involved in their development. However, most of the hypotheses are drawn from clinical work with adults. It is assumed that children who show symptoms of anxiety also over-react to threatening situations, have little confidence in their coping ability and will tend to report catastrophizing thoughts and worries.

Prins (2001) reviewed some of the recent research on cognitive-behavioural and information processing approaches. The cognitive-behavioural model relies on self-report and stresses the role played by negative belief systems in the onset and development of anxiety disorders. Cognitive schemas which become dysfunctional provide the basis for biased interpretations of external events. This distorts the information that is stored in schemas, the cognitive content. Distortion can also take place in the process of interpreting external events and inferring meaning through attending disproportionately to threatening cues. Conscious thoughts and images are the cognitive products which can result in negative self-talk and negative thoughts.

The cognitive-behavioural theory of childhood anxiety assumes that anxiety disorders result from chronic overactivity of schemas organized round themes of threat and danger, focusing processing resources on threat-relevant information (Kendall and Ronan, 1990). As they grow older children can increasingly make themselves anxious through their own thinking, but can also learn to cope cognitively with anxiety. An important issue here is whether 'coping cognitions' help or hinder anxious children's behaviour. Vasey and Daleiden (1996) described two pathways of cognitive interference in anxious children. Firstly, there are attentional processes early in the sequence that may stimulate children's anxiety. Secondly, attempts to cope with the threatening situation and with the anxiety itself use up processing resources and may interfere with their efforts to cope. A number of authors refer to the observation that children with high anxiety report more negative cognitions and more coping self-talk. The assumption underlying the use of cognitive-behavioural approaches with selectively mute children has been that negative cognitions and self-talk characterize their image of themselves as social beings. Spence, Donovan and Brechman-Toussaint (2000) have demonstrated that cognitive-behavioural therapy can be effective in the treatment of social phobia in childhood. A particular initiative in the treatment of selective mutism has been the use of self-modelling within a cognitive-behavioural theoretical framework.

The starting point for work on self-modelling was Bandura's (1977) idea of 'self-efficacy'. He argued that all procedures to change behaviour are effective to the extent that they modify the individual's perception of their own efficacy or competence. This would acknowledge that the person has the necessary skills in their repertoire to act effectively, but fails to do so. He described therapy as 'changing partly the acquisition of coping skills and also the acquisition of a self-belief that one can successfully execute the behaviour required'. For these reasons it was predicted that the use of self-modelling would be more powerful than the use of peer models. Both peer modelling and self-modelling have been used by Gelfand (1979) in the treatment of children's fears and by several therapists using edited videotape with selectively mute children. Dowrick and Hood (1978) used it in an elegant study with two selectively mute children. The authors were able to show that each child only changed his behaviour when he watched a tape of himself and not when he watched a tape of the other child. It seems likely that, as they watch the faked videotape of themselves talking normally in a classroom situation, the children learn to believe that they really can act like that. It is then only a short step to do so in the actual situation. (For a fuller account of how these videotapes were made, see Appendix 3.)

The cognitive perspective that influenced those initiatives has also had an impact on how 'reward' is conceived. Lepper and Gilovich (1981) differentiated between the following effects of reward – acting as an incentive, exerting social control, and providing social feedback on performance. Much work in the behavioural tradition emphasizes the first two of these effects; theorists adopting this perspective emphasize the third. They highlight the importance of intrinsic motivation which comes from feeling competent and feeling that one has autonomy and choice. The informational aspects of reward are seen as having a crucial influence on intrinsic motivation. It is not enough that people recognize that they have done what is required and met some criterion of successful performance. If they are to change their behaviour after this experience, they must also come to believe that the achievement was attributable to themselves: **they** did it (Deci and Ryan, 1985). Extrinsic rewards of one kind or another may be effective as an incentive for most people, but they do not convey that crucial message. In fact external rewards may lessen intrinsic motivation for an activity, because people may perceive that they only did it because of something outside themselves. These ideas have been applied widely to the challenges of school life (Wright, 1991). Their particular relevance for selective mutism was discussed by Lachenmeyer and Gibbs (1985) whose work with Joey was described in Chapter 4.

Historical outline

For convenience the material has been divided under four main headings:

- naive and eclectic use of behavioural approaches
- early applications of behaviour therapy up to 1971

- later case reports 1971–1981
- advances in the application of behavioural principles 1982–2002.

Naive and eclectic use of behavioural approaches

'Naive and eclectic use' is taken to include both the occasional use of behavioural methods by therapists holding a psychodynamic view of selective mutism and its intuitive use by parents, teachers and others.

Parents and teachers have always used behavioural techniques with difficult children, and the case histories of selective mutes are full of examples of naive behavioural approaches often quoted to emphasize the intractability of the problem. Sharon's father 'tried two opposite approaches at different times: at one time he used bribery, offering Sharon a variety of fantastic gifts if she would speak. At other times. . . . he would badger her unmercifully with a great deal of yelling and screaming' (Crema and Kerr, 1978). Of Susie the referring doctor wrote: 'The muscular tic began in March 1968 following a period when, at the suggestion of the school psychologist, the parents were using withdrawal of food for several days, . . . and other methods for forcing her to talk' (Dmitriev and Hawkins, 1973). Teachers, too, have tried to manage the problem through reward and punishment. Shaw (1971) described the case history of Wilma, a girl from a Dutch family who had emigrated to Canada. Wilma's older sister was said to have been electively mute at school for a time. 'This behaviour was forcibly terminated by corporal punishment at school.' Wilma too was persistently silent at school, though making normal academic progress. She was physically punished at least twice for this at school with no effect.

Some therapists, who present their clients in psychodynamic terms, have employed behavioural methods. For example, Youngerman (1979) described a selectively mute 14-year-old in an inpatient clinic who was not given his weekend pass to go home unless he asked for it aloud. Increasing demands were made so that each time he had to say more. Koch and Goodlund (1973), who used psychotherapy combined with parental counselling, mentioned that 'reward systems' were used with three children (in conjunction with loss of privileges unless these were requested verbally). Reviewing the literature from a psychodynamic perspective, Ruzicka and Sackin (1974) comment: '. . . even dynamically oriented therapists seem to take on a behaviouristic orientation when confronted with the electively mute child.'

Intuitively some therapists have arrived at variants on behavioural techniques designed to generalize children's speech once it had been elicited in a one-to-one situation. For example, Smayling (1959), a speech therapist, used a version of stimulus fading when she helped case F, an intelligent boy with a long history of mutism, transfer his oral reading to the classroom. (See also the use of a similar strategy by another speech therapist – Strait, 1958.) Landgarten (1975), whose art therapy approach is fully described in Chapter 5, took care to introduce Cora, once speech had been established, to other people working in the clinic.

Other writers saw the usefulness of behaviour therapy in schools, although they were writing from a psychodynamic perspective. An interesting example of this is the review by Halpern, Hammond and Cohen (1971). They recommended behavioural methods, although conceptualizing selective mutism in psychodynamic terms. They saw what they called 'partial speech avoidance' as a defence to protect the child's self-image 'arising out of an overvaluation by the child of his own power'. The children were described (with reference to Thomas, Chess and Birch, 1968) as temperamentally slow to warm up, having intrapsychic concerns about the inferiority or weakness of their voices and compensating for this by maladaptive coping behaviour. They compared elective mutism to school phobia and felt that it needed similarly prompt treatment, describing the therapist as the 'master strategist' in formulating tactics to get the child to speak in school. The suggested intervention appears to be escape/avoidance. It is first discussed carefully with parents and teachers. The plan is explained to the child the day before, in the presence of the class. At the end of the school day the child has to speak one pre-selected word before being allowed to go home. Subsequently the tariff is raised until 'more or less normal performance is achieved'. Two cases were described in some detail, one of a 7-year-old boy and another of 6-year-old twins. Not surprisingly, only limited speech seems to have been obtained. However, Halpern and his colleagues saw the need to involve parents and teachers fully in the consultation stage and anticipated the possible anxieties which might arise, as well as the need to continue the same approach until speaking was established.

A particular concern of workers with a psychodynamic orientation using common-sense behavioural approaches is the possibility of symptom substitution: the child will talk satisfactorily, but underlying problems will not have been resolved, and new emotional or behavioural difficulties will develop in the place of the mutism. Halpern, Hammond and Cohen (1971) formulated their reassurance on this point in psychodynamic terms: 'if the child can be shown how to gain rational mastery over the phobic situation he is in a better position to strengthen those controlling functions of the ego which moderate drives and effects.' (p. 105) Reviewing the literature 12 years later, Hesselman (1983) commented that few psychoanalytic theorists were actually critical of behaviour therapy. Referring to concerns expressed by some writers about the possibility of symptom displacement she argued that there was no evidence for this.

Early applications of behaviour therapy up to 1971

The first substantial paper to explore in detail the application of behavioural approaches to selective mutism was the review by Reed (1963). He aimed to tackle the questions of aetiology and treatment in an ambitious linked discussion which had a considerable influence. In his four cases he had not found the common pattern of background factors reported by some earlier writers such as Salfield (1950) and Morris (1953). Although agreeing that they presented some similar behavioural features, he argued that his cases represented at least two clinical sub-types – the attention-seeking, negativistic type and the more phobic, timid one. He felt the behaviour might be the outcome of a variety of drives operating in different personality types. Therefore a standard approach to treatment was unlikely to be successful and should not be recommended. Treatment was to be based on relearning, as the first group had acquired mutism as an avoidance tactic which gained attention, whereas the second group had developed it as a fear-reducing mechanism. For the attention-seeking group he suggested that the mutism should be ignored, while building up their self-esteem by a focus on other aspects of their appearance and behaviour. The timid type should have therapy designed to establish rapport and diminish fear, followed by attempts to generalize new behaviours to other settings in the clinic, and then to other adults, and finally to groups of children and adults. Here the cooperation of home and school would be important – to widen by easy stages the number and types of safe situations.

Reed's article has obvious limitations – he based the 'sub-types' model on a very small number of subjects and failed to give clear details about treatment. Nonetheless it has often been quoted and has subsequently influenced many workers to make a distinction between timid and manipulative selective mutes. Key factors in the continuing popularity of Reed's ideas are the paradoxical and, in some cases, even bold and aggressive nature of the children's behaviour and the effect of unsuccessful treatments which seem to strengthen the mutism. Where selective mutism is thought of exclusively as an acquired fear, it is hard to include in the category those children who had established rewarding systems of non-verbal communication in school and who had not responded to sympathetic and gentle handling. The continuing strength of the influence of Reed's distinction may be seen in papers as recent as Lumb and Wolff (1988).

Other early studies used the operant model of behaviour which made no assumptions about causes or about distinctions between personality types but simply described, measured and recorded behaviour. Straughan, Potter and Hamilton (1965) applied a technique which had been used by other psychologists to modify hyperactive behaviour in the classroom, linking reward to the activation of a signal light and counter and in addition using peer group approval as a social reinforcer. 'Presumably peers are much more reinforcing than therapists,' wrote Straughan in comparing his case to Reed's. (The scarcity of published studies at that time can be noted, as Reed's is the only reference Straughan et al. made to case reports on selective mutism.) They acknowledged that their subject, Gene (aged 14), had some baseline speech in the classroom preceding the intervention. For their approach to succeed some baseline speech is necessary. (This case is also discussed briefly in Chapter 7.)

In another paper Straughan (1968) discussed the difficulty of obtaining generalization and maintenance of changes in the children's speech. He suggested that a therapist should consider 'preparing or changing the social environment to support and encourage speech when it does occur'. Here he had in mind the need to reward changes in peer group behaviour when what peers do is being used as a source of reinforcement.

Studies using operant techniques to elicit or increase speech or vocalization in children who were preverbal or with very limited speech were comparatively numerous at this period, e.g. Cook and Adams (1966). These children would now not be described as selectively mute. For example, Blake and Moss (1967) also used a visual feedback system, a 'colour organ' in a special teaching booth, in work with a non-verbal child, Dolly (aged 4). The first step was to elicit eye contact and compliance, followed by imitation of both non-verbal behaviours and vocalization. This case study incorrectly uses the term 'electively mute' in its title and has often been cited in the literature for that reason. In fact Dolly did not speak at all at the outset and could not be described as selectively mute within the definition set out in Chapter 1. The application of operant techniques to eliciting speech from children with severe learning difficulties has continued to influence even recent work (e.g. Pecukonis and Pecukonis, 1991). In certain cases these approaches may serve to elicit speech initially. (See Chapter 7 for a discussion of the situations when this approach is most useful.) Unfortunately, many of these approaches focus on artificial speech responses and do not make use of the normal speech which is in the selectively mute child's repertoire. For this reason, perhaps, the process takes an excessively long time and the outcome sometimes falls short of spontaneous speech.

Some of the early case studies, which are mainly anecdotal and make no attempt at single case experimental design, still repay close reading because of the honesty with which they describe the therapist's attempts to provide effective help. As noted above, there were few references to which workers in this period could turn for constructive advice, as the literature still generally described the problem as 'intractable.' But much can still be learned from the careful observations some of these workers made. For example, Brison (1966) gave an illuminating retrospective account of work with Tom (aged 6). He had not spoken in his first kindergarten year and therefore had to repeat the year. Six months later he had still not spoken in school. The psychologist had seen Tom several times both on his own and in classroom observation, and there had been discussions with his teachers and parents and the district speech consultant. Tom and his family lived in an isolated area, and his parents said he spoke little to his grandparents, and to local children only if their mother was not present. Referrals were made to an audiologist, to a paediatrician and to a psychiatrist. The latter viewed Tom's behaviour as the manifestation of an underlying emotional disturbance, believing that the behaviour could not be treated directly because of symptom substitution. When the parents did not accept the psychiatrist's recommendation of psychotherapy, an alternative plan had to be made, because Tom was reacting adversely to his kindergarten teacher's strenuous attempts to get him to talk to her. Tom was moved to another class for the last weeks of term where no reference was made to his lack of speech, although the teacher reinforced his non-verbal communication. After the summer holiday she gradually stopped reinforcing this and did not attend to his non-verbal signs. Soon after this Tom began to talk, first on the school bus and in the playground, then in the classroom 'in an off-stage whisper', and then directly with his teacher. He did well in his school work, and no further problems were found on follow-up 3 years later.

Brison admitted that he only arrived at the final behavioural treatment plan intuitively and that he saw *post hoc* that Tom's non-speaking could be analysed in terms of learned behaviour which could be changed through the systematic manipulation of contingencies. With hindsight, Brison mentioned alternatives which would have been more rapidly effective, including involving Tom's parents in 'systematic desensitization by getting him to talk in a progressive series of situations leading to speech in the classroom.' He also mentions the possibility of Tom listening to recordings of his own voice, first in an empty classroom and then with other children present. Brison was sensitive to the distress caused to Tom, his teacher and his parents and the way in which his failure to speak produced responses from others that added to his difficulties. 'In short, the consequences of not treating the symptom were dire.' This report contains one of the first suggestions that tape-recorders could be used to help selectively mute children.

Reid et al. (1967) and Sluckin and Jehu (1969) are good examples of therapists' effective use of operant techniques, including stimulus fading. Reid's study illustrates the rapidity with which speaking can be transferred to other situations and people. Sluckin and Jehu describe a more lengthy process of intervention but refer explicitly to the operant techniques used. Both reports will be discussed fully in the next chapter because there are lessons for practice now in their detailed description of what the therapists did and the degree to which they involved parents in the work with their child.

Later case reports 1971–1981

In the decade from 1971 there were still some anecdotal reports of the casual application of behavioural principles (e.g. Inniss, 1977), but there were also signs of the development of a more systematic approach. Most importantly, a number of authors attached reviews to case reports on a group of children, usually those referred to a single child psychiatric clinic or in a single district over a period of years. Among these are Friedman and Karagan (1973) and Kolvin and Fundudis (1981). These reviews mainly cover issues such as aetiology, incidence and characteristics of the children. They also discuss methods of treatment or intervention, but usually with little detail. There were, however, important reviews of methodology by Sanok and Ascione (1979), Kratochwill, Brody and Piersel (1979), and Kratochwill (1981). In this 10-year period there was a marked increase in the number of published reports of all kinds on selective mutism, both case studies and some single subject experimental designs.

In 1973 a report by Calhoun and Koenig described a controlled group study of eight 'selectively mute' children with a positive outcome for the experimental group using positive reinforcement and extinction of non-verbal response. However, it is clear that the children who were the subject of this study already had a low level of speech in the classroom at the out-set and could not be correctly described as selectively mute. In the same year Wulbert et al. produced a good example of a single case experimental design, and there were further reports on successful outcomes in 1974 from Bednar and from Rasbury. In that year too Conrad, Delk and Williams highlighted the contribution of cultural differences to selective mutism, introducing a theme that was to reappear increasingly frequently in the lit-erature on intervention. They suggested that, when a child is from an ethnic or linguistic minority community, it is important to use workers from the same community in work with the child (see Chapter 7).

In a significant paper Brown, Fuller and Gericke (1975) questioned the claims for the effectiveness of behavioural approaches that were being made in the literature. They pointed out that almost all reports were of sin-gle cases only, using approaches with most of the features of systematic desensitization with clear-cut success. They suggested that so far only Reed's 'phobic mutes' had appeared in the published cases, and they argued that reports describing unsuccessful outcomes were needed. The child they described was Ian who had first been referred to a psychologist at age 5 because he did not speak in school. A year in an educational ther-apy unit had no effect, and he was referred to a child psychiatry clinic when he was 8. His family relationships and early history of shyness were fully described. Ian did not speak in playgroup or in infant or junior school. Significantly Ian's parents had 'tried all manner of common-sense tactics to encourage him to speak – mainly coaxing, but also coercion.' Observation indicated that Ian's mutism was being maintained both at home and at school, as one of his brothers and a child in his class constantly interpreted his needs. No less than three formulations of the problem were made.

- Ian was seen as phobic, reducing his anxiety by physical withdrawal or removal of eye contact. For 11 sessions the two therapists played games with Ian at his home in a desensitization approach. There was some reinforcement using modelling straws that Ian loved as a reward. Although Ian appeared to enjoy the games, his responses were unpre-dictable and no progress seemed to be made.
- A second formulation was made of latent aggression, i.e. that Ian was withdrawing from situations at home and at school in order to assert himself. The next 17 sessions encouraged aggressive and verbally

expressive responses through a range of activities in the clinic with a variety of reinforcers offered for even approximations in the direction of expressive speech such as shaking his head in appropriate situations or increasing eye contact. Ian's play became more aggressive and eye contact did increase, but he did not speak. It was felt that Ian was enjoying the positive attention and gaining control over the therapists' behaviour rather than the reverse.

• This led to a third 'control' formulation of the problem and one final 'marathon' session at the clinic with close control over Ian's environment. The idea was that during this session he would only gain access to things he wanted by making progressive approximations to verbal contact. The criterion of what response was required in order to obtain play materials or food was steadily made more challenging. By the end of 8 hours Ian had made few responses, though he had reached a level where he had to press the buzzer and say one word. The therapists thought that even if the session continued until he made further approximations to speech, Ian's controlling behaviour would persist. It was felt to be ethically wrong to extend the level of control over Ian and a waste of time and resources to continue. The therapists were tempted to wonder whether resistant cases of elective mutism should be tackled by default and the children 'allowed to grow out of it.'

It is important to encourage the publication of cases with unsuccessful outcomes, but this case study is also valuable in illustrating how much harder it is to work successfully with a child with whom many ineffective attempts at intervention have already been tried. Other workers have shown that in such cases it is usually necessary to employ a combination of operant techniques, including response cost. (An example of an effective intervention package with an older child may be found in Sanok and Striefel, 1979.)

In 1977 Sluckin published another case report, extending her earlier work, and Williamson et al. (1997a, 1997b) published two important reports, each dealing with two single experimental designs. These, with Scott (1977) and Richards and Hansen (1978), are described in Chapter 7. Crema and Kerr (1978) provided another example of a report in which therapists reflected constructively on setbacks in a process of intervention that was eventually successful. It can again be seen with hindsight that the process could have been speeded up if the early stages of treatment had been based on a systematic assessment of the child's situation and behaviour.

Advances in the application of behavioural principles 1982–2002

Earlier reviews by Labbe and Williamson (1984) and Cunningham et al. (1983) tabulated reports of behavioural work with selective mutism under a set of overlapping headings. We have used the headings common to both these reviews and incorporated most of those used by Kratochwill (1981) in a tabulation of most work between 1982 and 2002 (Table 6.2).

Table 6.2 Reports of behavioural approaches 1982–2002

Authors	Sex	Age (years)	Design	Techniques	Outcome (level of speech, generalization)	Follow-up
Afnan and Carr (1989)	F	6	Case study	Stimulus fading, family work and play	Reported fluent in all settings	No
Albert-Stewart (1986)	M[a]	13	Case study	Positive reinforcement use of tape-recorder	Improved volume and intelligibility	No
Barlow, Strother and Landreth (1986)	F	5	Case study	Play therapy with sibs (stimulus fading)	Spontaneous speech in clinic; reported progress in school	No
Bayley and Hirst (1991)	F	6	Case study	Positive reinforcement with some confrontation	Speech generalized to a range of settings in school	No
Bozigar and Hansen (1984)	4 F	6–9	Case study	Group therapy (response elicitation, stimulus fading)	Spoke in new schools; more spontaneous at home	3, 6, 12 months later
Brown and Doll (1988)	F[a]	6	Case study	(a) Reinforcement for whole class	Peer-directed speech, low volume	6 months later
				(b) Individual reinforcement in three phases (incl. use of voice light) and withdrawal	Increase in volume with reinforcement, token system and voice light	3 months later
Clayton (1981)	F	6	Systematic case study	Response elicitation and stimulus fading	Spontaneous speech at school; reported better at home	9 months later

Table 6.2 Reports of behavioural approaches 1982–2002

Authors	Sex	Age (years)	Design	Techniques	Outcome (level of speech, generalization)	Follow-up
Croghan and Craven (1982)	F	8	Case study	(a) Positive reinforcement and response cost (b) Desensitization	Limited speech to one teacher and two friends Spoke to staff and pupils	15 months later 6 months later
Cunningham et al. (1983)	(a) M (b) M	3 15	Single-case experimental design Single-case experimental design	Stimulus fading of teacher, then peers into family play Shaping and positive reinforcement and stimulus fading	Spoke to teachers and then peers in the classroom Spontaneous, audible speech gradually extended	6 months later 1, 2 months later
Giddan et al. (1997)	F	8	Case study	Response initiation; stimulus fading; shaping; contingency management; cross-site transfer	Now speaks with ease at school and in the community	No
Gupta (1990)	F	6	Case study	Successive approximation; stimulus fading; confrontation	Success achieved only after a change of school	3 months later
Hill and Scull (1985)	M[a]	9	Case study	Positive reinforcement and turn-taking games	More speech and increased activity generally	Over 4-year period
Holmbeck and Lavigne (1992)	F	6	Case study	Self-modelling, stimulus fading and contingency management	Talking freely with therapist after 8 sessions and in school from session 13	6 months later
Imich (1987)	F	4	Case study	Systematic desensitization	Speaking easily in classroom and playground	6 months later

Table 6.2 Reports of behavioural approaches 1982–2002

Authors	Sex	Age (years)	Design	Techniques	Outcome (level of speech, generalization)	Follow-up
Kehle, Owen and Cressy (1990)	M	6	Case study	Self-modelling, edited video, positive reinforcement	Normal speech in all settings after second videotape	7 months later
Larsson and Larsson (1983)	(a) F[a]	6	Single-case experimental design	Stimulus fading with single peer	Verbal compliance in group reading. Improved response to different questions. Some spontaneous speech	No
	(b) F[a]	11	Single-case experimental design	Multiple baseline, fading in one peer at a time	As for (a)	No
Lazarus, Gavillo and Moore (1983)	(a) F	6	Case study	Response elicitation, reinforcement, stimulus fading (with rabbit, puppets)	Spoke to teacher, child and small group	No
	(b) F	7	Case study	Stimulus fading from family therapy setting to school	Reading and spontaneous speech to psychologist, teacher, peers	Rest of school year, next year
Lindblad-Goldberg (1986)	M	5	Case study	Family therapy and stimulus fading with reinforcement for successive approximations. Used phone/puppets/games	Spoke to stepfather, then grandfather, then therapist and teacher in family meetings at clinic. Led to stimulus fading in school	24 months later
Lumb and Wolff (1988)	(a) F	5	Case study	Response elicitation and stimulus fading	Spoke to friend, teachers, then in class	6 months later

Table 6.2 Reports of behavioural approaches 1982–2002

Authors	Sex	Age (years)	Design	Techniques	Outcome (level of speech, generalization)	Follow-up
Lumb and Wolff (1988)	(b) F	11	Case study	Response cost and stimulus fading	Verbal compliance and some spontaneous speech	End of next term
Lysne (1995)	M	14	Case study	Contingency management; escape procedure	Within 2 weeks able to speak like everyone else at school and in his social life	No
Masten et al. (1996)	M	8	Case study	Shaping; stimulus fading	Speaking in therapy settings but no generalization to classroom	No
Morin, Ladouceur and Cloutier, (1982)	M[a]	6	Single-case experimental design	Positive reinforcement ABABB design	Increased frequency of response in class	12 months later
Paniagua and Saeed (1987)	F	11	Single-case experimental design	Response elicitation, positive reinforcement and response cost	Increase in some elicited speech about pictures	No
Pecukonis and Pecukonis (1991)	M	7	Single-case experimental design	Positive reinforcement to train non-verbal attending, verbal imitation and language	Non-verbal attending and verbal imitation above criterion but not functional language	No
Pigott and Gonzales (1987)	M	7	Systematic case study	Self-modelling on edited video played at home. Self-monitoring and reinforcement added	Increased rate of answering questions; ambiguous result on volunteering answers; increase after reinforcement	6 months later

Table 6.2 Reports of behavioural approaches 1982–2002

Authors	Sex	Age (years)	Design	Techniques	Outcome (level of speech, generalization)	Follow-up
Porjes (1992)	1F, 1M	6	Case studies	Ecological analysis; compiling a reinforcement menu; contingency management	Both children speak in all required situations in school, though in one case only quietly	No
Powell and Dalley (1995)	F	6	Case study	Family advice, stimulus fading, audio self-modelling, play therapy	Generalization of speaking to a range of people and settings	6 months later
Richburg and Cobia (1994)	F	5	Case study	Contingency management; stimulus fading	Speaking to teacher in front of class – even after change of class	No
Sheridan, Kratochwill and Ramirez (1995)	F	6	Single-case experimental design	Problem analysis; response initiation procedures; peer prompting; stimulus fading	Stimulus fading led to her speaking to eight individuals across three school settings	None after end of school year
Watson and Kramer (1992)	M	9	Single-case experimental design	Shaping, multiple reinforcers, stimulus fading, mild aversives. Separate regimes at home and school	Home results positive – increased frequency; spoke in new settings. School progress not maintained or generalized	3 month intervals
Weckstein, Krohn and Wright (1995)	2 M	6, 7	Case studies	Hawthorn Center approach (see Chapter 8)	Substantial improvements at school and within the family	No

Table 6.2 Reports of behavioural approaches 1982–2002

Authors	Sex	Age (years)	Design	Techniques	Outcome (level of speech, generalization)	Follow-up
Winter (1984)	M[a]	7	Systematic case study	Non-verbal communication ignored. Positive reinforcement for speech from staff and peers. Reinforcement faded	Increase in speech, including spontaneous speech. Improved performance on test of expressive language	12 months later
Wright et al. (1985)	1 F, 2 M	4, 5	Case study	Reinforcement in nursery, closely involving parents	Began to talk to one staff member in outside play (2/3 cases)	No

[a] Child with baseline speech; 'reluctant talker'.

The advantages of behavioural strategies in general were now well established and were repeatedly confirmed in the few reviews that were published (see below) and in rare follow-up studies (e.g. Sluckin, Foreman and Herbert, 1991). During this period major advances were made in clarifying which specific behavioural approaches were most effective in different situations. For example, there was a clearer recognition that simpler techniques could be used for children who show some level of baseline speech but who still had some difficulties, perhaps with audibility. These simpler techniques often involve reinforcement for peers of the target child. Six reports on 'reluctant talkers' in the table illustrate this trend (Morin, Ladouceur and Cloutier, 1982; Larsson and Larsson, 1983; Winter, 1984; Hill and Scull, 1985; Albert-Stewart, 1986; Brown and Doll, 1988).

In two reports in which play or group therapy was the main intervention as seen by the authors (Bozigar and Hansen, 1984; Barlow, Strother and Landreth, 1986), a close reading of what happened suggests that stimulus fading was in fact the key component in the children's progress in that setting. These reports have therefore been included in the table.

Stimulus fading was an important component in all the case studies where work with the child's family was a feature, e.g. in the first case reported in Cunningham et al. (1983). In Lindblad-Goldberg (1986) it was skilfully combined with family therapy, and in Afnan and Carr (1989) the child's mother initiated its use. As noted elsewhere, when Croghan and Craven (1982) reviewed the 5-year history of work with JB, they concluded that 'had stimulus fading been introduced at the very beginning of treatment, her progress would have been much more rapid'. Again, the family had themselves used a similar technique to help JB talk to her new stepfather – an example of how professionals can learn from parents. (A comparison may be made with the report by Rasbury, 1974.) The only example of stimulus fading used in a controlled single case design with a child who was selectively mute in the target setting is that of Cunningham and co-workers. The authors make it clear that in their view this would be the intervention of choice with a young child.

Three interesting reports combine self-modelling on edited videotapes with peer reinforcement and some element of stimulus fading (Pigott and Gonzales, 1987; Kehle, Owen and Cressy, 1990; Kehle et al., 1998). As described in Chapter 4, the videotapes appeared to show the children answering questions from their teachers. Actually they were edited from footage of the teachers asking prepared questions (to which the child had not in fact answered) and the child answering the same questions (when put by their parents). Both children were apparently willing to speak with their families in front of the therapists in order to make the tapes. Because the next stage of intervention took place in the target setting of the classroom, there is some credibility in the claim that these are time-saving procedures.

In some reports intervention appears to start in a school or clinic setting without any recorded discussion of the possibility of involving members of the child's family or friends in treatment. Because the child is mute in these settings, it follows that intervention has to start with response initiation, e.g. Lazarus, Gavillo and Moore (1983) and Lumb and Wolff (1988). This is also true of the report by Clayton (1981), although in that case the psychologist involved Clarissa's friends at an early stage. Where such interventions begin with a figure who is unfamiliar to the child, they often take much longer, and generalization is then delayed (e.g. Masten et al., 1996). Some workers have gone through a period of unsuccessful treatment based on response initiation with 'strangers' and then made immediate progress when a member of the child's family became involved and a stimulus fading strategy was introduced (e.g. Sheridan, Kratochwill and Ramirez, 1995).

Response initiation procedures have often been combined with other procedures. Most reports of the use of a response initiation procedure describe work with older children of school age, some of them children who had been selectively mute for some time and with whom other interventions had been tried unsuccessfully (e.g. Paniagua and Saeed, 1987; Pecukonis and Pecukonis, 1991). However, there appears to be less likelihood of obtaining spontaneous speech at the end of treatment in such cases (see Table 6.2). Of course, spontaneous speech must be the ultimate goal if there is to be what Kratochwill would call a 'socially valid' outcome. Thus, further steps (including stimulus fading) need to be added in order to ensure generalization. These points are fully covered in the review paper by Labbe and Williamson, and are discussed in some detail in the next chapter.

Methodology

In all forms of treatment and intervention, practitioners agree that it is important to evaluate effectiveness. In his preface Kratochwill (1981) described the methodology of behaviour therapy as a sophisticated technology for measuring clinical change. However, his review of behavioural approaches to selective mutism showed that half the published reports were case study investigations which did not show that the intervention was responsible for the change in behaviour that was reported. He expressed the hope that practitioners would progress to better controlled interventions, making use of appropriate single case designs. Three other major reviews of behavioural work with selective mutism were published at around the same time as Kratochwill's – Sanok and Ascione (1979), Cunningham et al. (1983), and Labbe and Williamson (1984). All four emphasized the importance of experimental design – though some reviewers have summarized clinical reports without reference to methodological rigour, e.g. Hultquist (1995). Arguably, if more investigators had followed Kratochwill's advice, the major lessons of the last two decades of work in this field would have been learned much earlier. A recent systematic review by Stone et al. (2002) has indicated that the quality of research design has not improved greatly over subsequent years.

Sanok and Ascione (1979) drew up a table reviewing 16 reports on two parameters – design and outcome. The outcome was rated as positive if the design showed clearly that there was a functional relationship between the treatment and a positive change in the child's behaviour. This was the case in seven reports. Equivocal outcomes were those in which a functional relationship could not be demonstrated because of methodological problems or because positive results failed to generalize. Some reports failed to demonstrate efficacy because of a failure to plan for generalization with reference to the level of speech or the type of reinforcement used. Others failed because of lack of direct follow-up measures. They listed their main criticisms of the procedures in most studies which resulted in ambiguous outcomes:

- These usually resulted from insufficiently precise behavioural assessment. Often investigators failed to identify the exact antecedent conditions under which speech occurred. This led to confusion in choice of subject. A common example has been working as though children are selectively mute when they do in fact speak in all situations, though not very much – 'reluctant talkers' (e.g. Calhoun and Koenig, 1973; Bauermeister and Jemail, 1975). Sanok and Ascione showed how this mistake could be avoided by using a simple but extremely useful frequency table for recording observations of where and how the child speaks. (Their table was the starting point for the work that led to the rather more complex grids that are presented in Chapter 7 and Appendix 1.)
- There was failure to use a multiple baseline. Sanok and Ascione contended that all case studies using a single subject only should use a multiple baseline design because it makes it possible to evaluate the effect of the interventions through observing the sequence of related changes. A multiple baseline can be:

    - measurement of several target behaviours (e.g. answers to different kinds of questions, such as open and closed questions)
    - measurement across behaviours (e.g. prompted and spontaneous speech)
    - measurement across settings (e.g. home, school, clinic).

- There was inadequate choice and specification before the intervention of the behaviours being measured (the dependent variables). Although a positive change in spontaneous speech is generally the aim, there should be agreement in advance about the specific objectives for each subject. Measurements should be made in the presence of different persons and at several points in time: before, during and after intervention, and again after an interval for follow-up.

Kratochwill reviewed reports under the following headings – measurements and observer variables, outcome criteria, design, generalization, and follow-up.

Measurement

Measurement should include direct assessment of speech (or its absence) across different situations in the child's natural environment. Continuous assessment allows the therapist to perceive patterns or trends in the data. Video and audio recording is particularly useful in recording speech in certain situations, such as the family home, that may be inaccessible to an observer. Observation of children's non-verbal behaviour in a variety of situations helps to establish whether they are generally isolated and withdrawn or whether they are outgoing and confident in situations where speech is not required.

In direct assessment observer reliability should be considered. Questions arise about possible bias and idiosyncrasy both during the process of observation itself, and during the recording of behaviour (e.g. coding of responses). Training observers and checking on observer reliability have been accepted practice in other applications of behavioural methods, but few reports in the area of selective mutism address these issues.

Multiple measurement may involve other response systems as well as behaviours, e.g. physiological measures and self-report. Physiological measures (e.g. of raised levels of stress) do not seem to have been used in work with selectively mute children, perhaps because they are too intrusive. Self-report has been used with one or two children retrospectively, after they have begun to speak normally in all situations, but so far little information appears to have been gained. Parents sometimes report comments made by their children about their mutism, but these are usually justifications in response to parental questioning.

Outcome criteria

Like Sanok and Ascione, Kratochwill (1981) drew attention to the importance of having a clear definition of outcome criteria. This definition should be socially valid as well as experimentally rigorous. In the evaluation of an intervention children's behaviour should be compared to that of their peers, addressing the question of whether their behaviour is now in the normal social range for their school or neighbourhood. Moreover, subjective evaluation of a child's behaviour should be requested from the people closest to the child to make sure that the improvement is significant in important areas of everyday life.

Design

In the early stages of behavioural research much can be gained from the case study method. But the introduction of experimental design is necessary if we are to be sure that any observed change in behaviour is due solely to a planned intervention and is not caused by some other factor. When it is not normally possible to study large groups of subjects, as in selective mutism, the most powerful strategy is to employ experimental design within single subject case studies (e.g. alternating treatment procedures to observe the effects of each). Kratochwill pointed out that few reports in the literature on selective mutism up to 1981 included a design of that kind.

Generalization

Methodological questions under this heading include: Was generalization of speech included in the intervention plan? Has the target behaviour, once achieved in some target settings, been assessed in other settings? If it has been assessed, was this through direct measures or indirect report?

Different behaviours vary in the degree to which they are likely to generalize and be maintained over time. The settings in which they occur may be important in their generalization and maintenance, often because natural social reinforcers are available. With selectively mute children the choice of intervention strategy may be another factor affecting both generalization and maintenance: it appears that when stimulus fading is used, either alone or in combination with other forms of intervention, generalization and maintenance may be secured without additional steps of intervention (Reid et al., 1967).

Follow-up

Follow-up should be included in any critical evaluation of behavioural approaches. Kratochwill expressed the view that it should be by direct measurement, not based on second-hand indirect report. He argued that it should be carried out at a minimum of two points in time, preferably soon after intervention has been completed and again after an interval.

Cunningham el al (1983) reviewed the published material and summarized 41 cases in a table. Only 6 were based on single case experimental designs from which conclusions could be made about treatment outcomes. Although 90% of the cases claimed follow-up, only two reports showed systematic behavioural data. Another matter for concern was that spontaneous speech was reported in 14 out of 18 case studies, but in only 1 out of 6 controlled single case designs. It could be argued that this implies a possible bias in reporting. An alternative explanation might be that stimulus fading is the procedure that appears least often in controlled experimental reports and is also the procedure most often associated with a successful outcome of spontaneous speech. Cunningham and his co-workers added to their review a report on two of their own cases, using controlled single case designs. The first was chosen to examine the effectiveness of stimulus fading procedures without reinforcement; the second used a combination of single case designs to see whether shaping and reinforcement could be used to produce speech in children who showed no baseline speech in the target setting. This report illustrated the value of establishing through the use of controlled studies the relative contribution of different procedures.

Labbe and Williamson (1984) grouped the case studies in their review of the literature according to the intervention or the combination of interventions. They emphasized the importance of careful assessment and suggested that the outcome of this should provide a clear rationale for choosing an intervention. Understanding of selective mutism would be demonstrated if therapists could make specific predictions about which intervention would best be used with each child and test this empirically.

How far were the methodological criticisms of these reviewers taken on board by those reporting on the treatment of selective mutism in the literature? An inspection of Table 6.2 shows that only 7 of the 33 reports summarized from the two decades that followed could clearly be described as having controlled experimental designs, although 3 others reported speech data that were collected at several points in time. Just over half of the studies (18) included follow-up, and this was often collected at second hand with no direct observations of the children. There is a tension between the interests of researchers and reviewers, seeking generalizable conclusions about a category of problems, and those of professional workers in a clinic or school setting, seeking an effective way of helping particular clients on particular occasions in the context of a heavy workload. The latter may have little motivation for the time-consuming observations and grandiose research designs that the former would like to impose on them. Some compromise between these two sets of interests was necessary if the progress reported in this chapter was to be continued in the future. The review by Stone et al. (2002) suggests that that has not been satisfactorily achieved. The final chapter of this book focuses on research design. The next chapter now builds on what was learned during the 30-year history of behavioural approaches to selective mutism. The benefits of employing behavioural methods in combination with other approaches are discussed in Chapter 8.

Chapter 7
Linking assessment and intervention

Over the period covered by the historical account in Chapter 6 it came to be accepted that intervention plans using behavioural approaches were the most effective treatments for the majority of children who are selectively mute. A combination of behavioural methods can often be matched to the individual needs of each child, sometimes in conjunction with other approaches. We show in the next chapter that there is now increasing interest in the possibility that psychopharmacology has a contribution to make in cases where other forms of intervention, including behavioural approaches, have proved ineffective. Combined approaches, for example of medication and behaviour therapy, are discussed in that chapter. But for most children who are selectively mute the debate is no longer about whether behavioural approaches should be used but how to use them most effectively, with particular reference to assessment and intervention.

When we wrote the first edition of this book 10 years ago the use of behavioural techniques was already widespread, and this in itself was an advance on the earlier use of psychodynamic approaches, which had focused on what were thought to be the historical causes of the behaviour. However, in many published case studies of behavioural treatment the choice of method seemed to be made on a trial and error basis. That is why our first principle was that, although many methods of intervention can be successful in some circumstances, the only way to ensure that the most effective and speedy method is used on each occasion is to base plans for intervention on a systematic assessment of the child's particular situation and, specifically, on the child's pattern of speaking and non-speaking behaviour. In behaviour therapy, assessment and intervention are reciprocal and continuous processes. Because there are usually many small steps in working with selectively mute children, assessment will be ongoing as the results of each stage are monitored.

The essential first step in matching intervention to children's needs is an analysis of all the circumstances in which they speak freely and those in which they do not. It is not always obvious to those who are accustomed to the child's pattern of communication why it is considered necessary to carry out this analysis in considerable detail. It is important to obtain information both from the people who know the child best and from those who are worried by the lack of speech in other situations. This usually includes the child's parents and teachers in school or nursery, but may also include members of the extended family.

Although there had been previous significant and important reviews of methodology, for example those by Sanok and Ascione (1979) and Kratochwill (1981), a major advance was made when Labbe and Williamson (1984) conducted a comparative analysis of case studies on an operant behaviour model. They suggested that there are five possible outcomes of a behavioural assessment of the settings in which a child speaks and that these can be linked to stages of intervention. We learned much from this model and adapted it as the basis of the staged procedure which we continue to find useful. The link can be shown to be hierarchical and ordered, so that assessment leads to stages of intervention, each building on the one before. Our adaptation of Labbe and Williamson's model is described in this chapter with a case study of Maria. Other case studies follow which have been chosen from the literature to illustrate how extensively the model applies.

That model is one of two major approaches to linking intervention and assessment that will be featured here. The other is entitled *functional analysis*. In this an attempt is made to identify functional relationships between events that occur regularly in a child's environment and aspects of the child's behaviour that are the target of attention. The fundamental question is asked – what factors trigger and maintain the pattern of behaviour that is seen as undesirable? A team of psychologists centred on the University of Wisconsin-Madison has investigated how principles of functional analysis might be applied to selective mutism (Sheridan, Kratochwill and Ramirez, 1995; Schill, Kratochwill and Gardner, 1996a, 1996b). The approach that they have evolved is described in the latter part of the chapter, and we suggest how these two approaches can complement each other in work with individual children, their families and schools.

In both approaches to intervention parents can play a key role in both assessment and treatment. This is widely acknowledged. What is not so apparent in most published studies is the need to be aware of the level of a child's anxiety. The failure to take this fully into account appears to be a frequent reason for setbacks when carrying out a programme. That is why anxiety and temperament have been extensively discussed in previous chapters. When there are indications that a child's anxiety level has risen to a point where progress is not possible, it may help to repeat the stage that has just been completed and reduce the size of each step that follows. It is then easier to discover what is making the present stage so difficult and making the child so anxious.

There are different views about the assessment of selectively mute children. The approach described here involves behavioural assessment that is designed to provide the basis for planning intervention. The core information is an analysis of the people and settings where the child does or does not speak, based on information from parents and those who know her best. Additional information from parents is also needed about her developmental history (especially in relation to speech and language skills), her temperament, and particular anxieties and fears. There are useful indirect measures which children can complete with their parents at home, for example Matson's fear thermometer (Matson, 1981). Information about speech and language skills can be gathered by a variety of means, including not only reports from those who hear her speak such as her parents but also from audio and video recordings (see Chapter 8). Some practitioners see the need for direct assessment of intellectual ability at this point. There are good reasons for thinking that this may be counterproductive, increasing children's level of anxiety and giving an inaccurate picture of their ability. With older children teachers can provide relevant information and produce examples of school work. With younger children much can be learned about their intellectual maturity by examining their drawings and paintings, observing their play at home or nursery and their response to books. If any formal assessments appear to be needed they should be carried out later when the child is speaking confidently. This chapter outlines a strategy that places less emphasis on information about a child's personality characteristics and greater emphasis on behavioural assessment and functional analysis that link more directly to the planning of intervention.

Involvement of parents in assessment and treatment

Many of the earlier case studies described the important insights contributed by parents during this process, and examples are included later in the chapter. Parents should be involved at all stages of assessment and treatment because of their intimate knowledge of the child and their capacity to contribute. In many cases one or both of them are the only people with whom she speaks freely. Almost always they are aware of the child's anxiety around aspects of speaking outside the home. Parents need to understand professionals' plans for the processes of assessment, which should start at the family home wherever possible because this is where the child will speak most freely.

For Maria (aged 4) the initial assessment at home and at nursery was based on the staged procedure derived from Labbe and Williamson that is described below. Assessment and intervention began at home where she was most comfortable speaking. This case underlined the importance of working closely with parents because they showed rapid understanding of the ideas underlying assessment and were able to contribute invaluable ideas to the planning of the programme of intervention. For example, near the end of the programme Maria's mother remembered the difficulty that her daughter had had at an early stage of assessment when more than one adult was introduced into the home at the same time. This was one of the factors that maintained her mutism in certain settings. As we will describe below, Maria started at a new school during the course of the intervention. At that point she could talk easily to adults, but to only one child. We planned a process of fading one child after another into situations at school where Maria spoke with adults. That proved unnecessary as her mother took the initiative and invited children home to play, but only one at a time. This enabled Maria to talk in school not only to children who had been to her home, but to other children as well. It also highlights the value of involving parents closely in the detailed assessment of the difficulties the child is experiencing and the step-by-step planning of any intervention. That will not always be possible but should always be attempted.

During the last 10 years or so parents have become more aware of selective mutism, mainly because of articles in newspapers and magazines, and more confident that their children can be helped. In some cases they have initiated referrals, sometimes through their family doctors, or nurseries and schools, and recently by making direct contact with psychologists and speech and language therapists. The development of parent support groups, for example the Selective Mutism Foundation Inc. in the USA and SMIRA in the UK (see Appendix 4), has encouraged them to seek help for their children, though in some areas it is still difficult to find. In some cases where the child is attending a setting outside home, the parents have already mentioned their anxiety to the staff and are ready for joint meetings and discussions.

Many referrals continue to come from schools or preschool settings, and when this happens it is essential for the psychologist or therapist to find out how the referral has been discussed with the child's parents and how the first contact with them should be made. Some parents find it easier to meet specialists at a school or nursery; others will choose a meeting at home at times when both parents can be present. In almost all cases it is preferable for the parents to be able to talk without the child (or any siblings) being present, and they may need some time in which to arrange child care. Those seeking to help a child who is referred for selective mutism should bear in mind the possibility that other members of the family, including one or both parents, may find initial contact with strangers intimidating.

In the initial meeting it may be possible to find out when the parents first noticed that the child spoke only to some people and in some settings, and to obtain some details of these settings and the children and adults spoken to by the child. Parents may be the best source of information about community settings where the child speaks outside the home. It is necessary to ask specifically about family, friends, neighbours, local shops, stores, park and playground, etc. (see the record grid for Maria below). The aide-mémoire for work with the family (Appendix 1) may help investigators to make sure that they cover the most important questions. It is of great value to give parents a copy of the record that is made of their views and observations, so that they can check that the record is accurate and can be shared with others.

Occasionally parents will say that the child talks a great deal at home, sometimes too much, but that nobody outside the family believes this. If they have made a tape of the child talking at home, this can be a useful source of information too, as well as suggesting a possible medium for later intervention. One use of such a tape may be to assess the quality of the child's speech and eliminate the possibility that articulation problems are contributing to their selective mutism (see Chapter 8). It is helpful also to ask whether the family have a video camera, or access to one, and to explain how this has been used in some cases to help children.

Parents may be reassured to know that their child's difficulties are shared by other children, and they are likely to find it helpful to be given a brief handout at the end of the discussion which explains the ways of helping children who are selectively mute and outlines the part that parents can play in the process. The handout should include contact phone numbers for the professionals involved and the address of a local or national support group if one is available. (See Appendix 4 for Internet sites that may be of value in this context.)

If the child is willing to talk to her parents, but not others, about her difficulty in speaking at school, they may be able to report what she has said. Of particular interest will be a list of the things that make her feel most anxious. It is equally important to know about her favourite activities and objects. This may help later in selecting rewards when planning a behavioural programme.

It may be helpful to mention to them that reward or reinforcement should not be limited to the tangible, often edible rewards so often described in reports of work using operant models. Kratochwill (1981) emphasized the importance of using natural social reinforcement whenever possible. Being able to talk to a wider circle of people brings its own satisfactions, as do the clear signs of parents' pleasure and approval. Before the child reaches that stage, planned social reinforcement may be effective. Examples in the literature have included additional private contacts with a teacher in school (Colligan, Colligan and Dillard, 1977) and playing a much enjoyed game (Furst, 1989). Alternatively, some workers have used more concrete or physical rewards that have had a social dimension because they encompassed other children, e.g. winning prizes on behalf of the whole class (Brown and Doll, 1988) and filling in a chart to earn a classroom party (Straughan, Potter and Hamilton, 1965). In addition, when the child is given some choice of reward or control over when and by whom it is given, the 'information' or feedback aspect of reward is highlighted, and the child is helped to acknowledge the achievement as his own (Lachenmeyer and Gibbs, 1985).

The parents may feel that immediate intervention is not really needed because they believe that the child will speak in time anyway or will speak when she has a different teacher. If they express such views, it may be necessary to describe the clinical evidence that supports an opposing view: that once a child has established selective mutism as a regular pattern of behaviour at school, she is unlikely to speak in school unless there is a systematic intervention to help her. Step-by-step stimulus fading usually makes sense to parents as a way of approaching the problem, when it is fully explained to them. That can lead on to a preliminary discussion of whether the best setting for this would be home or school.

Parents' permission should be obtained to observe the child in a setting where she does not speak. This may be done by the special educational needs coordinator (SENCO), by another teacher in the school, by a psychologist or speech and language therapist, to learn to what extent non-verbal communication is reinforced by teachers and by other children. (If there are plans for someone to work with the child at home it is often better if that person does not carry out the observation because some children seem to regard anyone whom they have seen at school as on the 'list' of people they do not speak to.)

It is essential to know what expectations the parents have of outside help, especially if attempts to persuade the child to talk have been made in the past and failed. It is important to make the aim of intervention explicit and to state it as simply and clearly as possible. For example, it might be to increase the number of situations where the child can speak freely and comfortably and to enable her to communicate normally in school. The aim will need to be agreed with all those involved. At this point we turn to another aspect of the assessment – the analysis of the situation at school.

Assessment at school

The child's teachers will be able to give a full educational history and a report on the child's adjustment on entry to school, her abilities and interests, temperament and personality. It will be important to ask what advice has been given in the past and who has already been consulted, both formally and through more unofficial channels (e.g. a teacher in another school who has taught a similar child). Was it possible to follow the advice and, if so, what were the results? It is useful to obtain as full an account as possible of all attempts to help the child and for how long they lasted. Earlier attempts at intervention, especially if they failed, are likely to have had an impact on the child and those around her, which will affect how they respond to a new initiative.

It is helpful to know how long she has been with the present teacher who will be able to say what strategies have been used to circumvent the mutism, for example in the literacy hour. Is she a lively child who often appears to be on the point of speaking, or is she passive, showing little expression? Does she ever laugh? Does she communicate if she hasn't understood something and if so how? Are there any activities which she will not take part in? Who are her friends, and have any of them taken on a special role which they may be unwilling to give up? (See Appendix 1 for other items.)

It is particularly valuable to talk with support staff who know the child well and may have worked with her in a small group. This creates particularly good opportunities for observation. They may also be able to give additional and useful information about the child's behaviour in the playground and other school settings and how she communicates with other children. They may mention times when she has been upset and come for help or identify activities which she seems to particularly enjoy.

Very often in school discussions in the past teachers would describe unsuccessful attempts to confront, coerce or trick the child into speaking, and negative feelings about the child's non-speaking would surface. In contrast to the situation 10 years ago when we prepared the first edition of this book, more teachers and support staff are now well informed about selective mutism. The prevailing reaction now seems to be anxiety that the child's difficulties should be resolved as soon as possible and sometimes frustration about delays or difficulties in obtaining help. Teachers' attitudes are often transformed when they understand that the children are anxious to a disabling degree, and that for some of them the only way of dealing with this is to show total resistance which may make them appear stubborn and obstinate. Some of the myths about selective mutism could be dealt with too, with a short explanation of how it develops. This discussion may be a crucial phase in laying the basis for planning effective intervention.

Making a visual record of an assessment of selective mutism

Communication and record keeping can be enhanced by the use of simple grids on which both preliminary and detailed assessments may be summarized. These have been adapted slightly over time, and we and other workers continue to use them as the basis for recording the outcomes of assessment and linking them to plans for intervention. One of the advantages of the grids is that they can be completed with parents and teachers who often contribute ideas for including additional settings and behaviour. They can also be updated to record the child's progress in new settings and with new people.

Table 7.1 Settings where Jane (aged 6) speaks

Speech	Setting		
	Home	School	Playground
Normal	*		
Low frequency		*	*
No speech			

This suggests that Jane is an 'infrequent speaker' rather than a selective mute. However, she will still need help to become more confident in settings outside the home. A programme might be used that offers positive reinforcement for speaking more often and more loudly.

The profile of a child with long-established selective mutism might look more like Elisabeth's in Table 7.2 below. This might require several stages of intervention using stimulus fading and positive reinforcement.

Table 7.2 Settings where Elisabeth (aged 6) speaks

Speech	Setting		
	Home	School	Playground
Normal	*		
Low frequency			*[a]
No speech		*	

[a] to one child only.

In order to plan intervention for a selectively mute child a more detailed analysis is needed, using information from indirect and direct sources. This is necessary to identify suitable points where stimulus fading might be introduced. This was discussed in detail in Chapter 6. We have illustrated it below by describing in detail the process of assessment and planning that was undertaken by one of us (SB) for one child (Maria). A more complex grid recording Maria's pattern of communication may be found there. As will be evident from that example, it is also possible to use the grids as a visual record of a child's progress, which can be employed not only to reward progress but also as the basis for discussing new targets. (Note that Johnson and Wintgens (2001) have developed a Talking Map which provides an excellent and age-appropriate way of involving a younger child in her own assessment.)

Case illustration of behavioural assessment and intervention – Maria

Maria (aged 4 years) had not spoken in her nursery class for a year, though she spoke to several family members at home and in one or two other settings. Maria was referred by the teacher in charge of the nursery class after she had tried a number of her own strategies to persuade Maria to speak and had discussed the problem with Maria's mother several times. At our initial meeting at school Maria's mother was rather distressed as she felt Maria's difficulties might have developed because she herself worked nights and sometimes left Maria watching television in the afternoons while she tried to catch up with her sleep. She also felt that nobody believed that Maria spoke normally at home. It was therefore reassuring to her when we started the discussion by making a detailed list of the situations where Maria did speak.

Table 7.3 Settings where Maria speaks

People	Places					
	Home	Aunt's	Church	Park	Shops	School
Mother	*	*	*	*	*	
Father	*	*		*		N/A
Aunt	*	*		*		N/A
Anna (cousin)	*	*		*		N/A
Marco (cousin)	*	*		*		N/A
Emma (friend)	*			*		*
Emma's mother	*			*		

This grid was used as the basis for discussion with Maria's family. Asterisks indicate where and with whom Maria normally spoke. As her father was never able to visit her nursery class, and her cousins attended a different school, the notation N/A was placed against their names for the school setting as the grid was not applicable to them in that setting.

The grid showed clearly that she spoke normally in some settings with a few people. Her parents strongly wished Maria's behaviour to change and, when stimulus fading was explained, welcomed it as a gradual approach which would take into account Maria's long-established shyness and what they described as her obstinacy. We discussed what would be the best setting for the first stage of intervention. Maria already spoke to a number of people in her home, her aunt's house and the park. Home was preferred by Maria's mother. The aunt's house was not suitable because her cousin Anna liked to speak for Maria, and this could have undermined the impact of the planned intervention. The park was ruled out as a possible setting because it was February. Maria spoke to Emma and her mother at her home, and sometimes walked home with them from school. The possibility of involving Emma in a school-based intervention was considered, but this was not pursued for two reasons: Emma had already gone up into the next class, and Maria was to attend a different school when she left the nursery class.

Maria was observed on three occasions for periods of 20 minutes in the nursery class. She made no verbal responses to any approaches from staff or children. She was also extremely passive, and showed no change in her facial expression to communicate understanding or feelings. She played alone and did not make any non-verbal approaches to other children, but would occasionally stand silently in front of an adult if she wanted something. She usually complied silently with the nursery routines, but never smiled or showed enthusiasm for any of the wide variety of activities available. Maria's teacher was most upset by her apparent inability to make choices and spent some time in each session trying to encourage Maria to take part. It was extremely difficult to resist doing this, although we both recognized that Maria was receiving a large amount of attention from adults that was reinforcing her mutism. Rewarding Maria with stickers for completed activities raised her activity level to some degree, but the effect was inconsistent.

A home visit was arranged. It was very clear that her mother wanted and expected Maria to talk to other adults, and had been angry and embarrassed when she remained silent on visits to other people's homes. Given firm cues by her mother, Maria began to speak to her and then to me about her dolls and other toys, but with reluctance. Her mother explained that as an only child Maria had a lot of attention from adults in the extended family, spending much of her day alone with her mother. She described Maria as extremely stubborn and very shy. There had been some difficulties at mealtimes because she disliked new foods.

Maria's mother is French and her father Spanish, and so two languages other than English are spoken in the home and at the aunt's house. Maria's father has a hearing impairment and speaks English with a heavy accent which she laughs at. Because of the family history of hearing difficulties and Maria's lack of response in settings outside the home (especially during visits to hospital outpatients), it was thought she might have a hearing loss. She failed a number of hearing tests and was fitted with a hearing aid which she hated and refused to wear. A specialist advisory teacher (WT) had also been asked to see Maria at home because of the concern about her behaviour in the audiology clinic. To the parents' relief we arranged to make joint visits. However, we found that if we visited separately Maria would speak to each of us in her mother's presence, but if we went together, she would say nothing. In retrospect, if we had employed functional analysis systematically at an early stage, we might have avoided this problem. We had noticed indications in the course of working with Maria that, when a number of people were present at the same time, she found it harder to speak and others were more likely to respond to her non-verbal signals. But, because we did not then use a functional analysis strategy in conjunction with our behavioural assessment, this point was missed in the planning of our intervention.

The same pattern was observed when the cousins and the aunt were invited to join Maria and her mother to play some board games with us at home. After initial reluctance, Maria began to join in, but did not speak except to count the spots on the dice for which she immediately received praise and a small reward. A video recording of these sessions shows clearly that at times we all (family members and visiting professionals) responded to Maria's non-verbal communication.

Because Maria talked so much at home, her mother was very willing to record her there on audio-tape. This gave good samples of her speech and showed that, although her language had normal, age-appropriate structures, her speech patterns resembled her parents' in intonation and rhythm (i.e. showing the influence of their first languages, French and Spanish). We also heard for ourselves that Maria knew most of the nursery rhymes she had been taught at school and enjoyed singing them.

Following this we planned that WT would continue to visit Maria at home once a week and would also see her at the nursery on a different day. Twice-weekly visits were time-consuming, but provided the opportunity for WT to carry out informal hearing tests in settings where Maria was more relaxed than in the hospital. We also made an experimental attempt, using stimulus fading, to see if she could begin speaking to WT in another setting – the nursery class. In the second week Maria began to whisper to WT there as long as nobody else was near enough to hear. If other children came closer she stopped speaking.

Up to this point we had concentrated on assessing Maria's speech in a variety of settings and with a variety of combinations of people, with increasing certainty that the outcome of the assessment pointed to stimulus fading and positive reinforcement as the intervention of choice. We planned a sequence of interventions to start at school after the Easter holiday in which other children and new adults would be gradually faded into those situations where Maria spoke with WT. However, a rapid change of plan had to be made when we heard just before the end of term that Maria had been offered early entry to her new school after Easter. As Maria's mother was expecting a second child in the summer, the parents thought that it would help Maria if she settled into her new school before the baby was born. A second unforeseen setback arose when we were told that WT's time with Maria would be cut as she was no longer thought to be severely hearing impaired because of the quality of her speech on the tape, including her responses to questions.

There were possible gains in the new situation because a change of school, especially when it occurs as a natural and desired progression, offers great advantages when working with selectively mute children. Stimulus control of speaking and not speaking has not been reinforced in the new school setting, and stimulus fading is easier to carry out in a setting where the child has not already got into the habit of withholding speech.

A meeting was arranged at the new school between the psychologist, the teachers and Maria's mother. Some of the teachers had heard about selective mutism, but none of them had direct experience of working with a selectively mute child. We played some of the tape of Maria singing and talking at home, and described the progress she had made. The teachers accepted her need for an introduction to school that would be gradual and would not raise her level of anxiety. They were also quick to pick up the importance of not reinforcing her non-verbal communication with attention and realized the difficulty they would have in doing this consistently.

The choice of stimulus fading as the preferred intervention was explained. One of the administrative staff, Lily, who came from the same language background as Maria's mother and attended the same church, offered to go back to the beginning of the process by visiting Maria at home. Once speech was established with Lily, the second step in the plan was to be a visit to school in the evening when no children would be there, perhaps just walking round the grounds. Because this was almost a repeat of a previous step, Maria spoke easily with her mother and Lily on the first visit, and they visited the school that evening, looking round the empty classrooms while Maria continued to talk. Two days later, Maria and her mother visited the school during the day and went with Lily to the reception classroom where Maria played with Lily and spoke to the teacher about a picture she had drawn. She also spoke to a second teacher in the playground ('My nursery has better toys than you have.') The teachers were extremely surprised, and in discussion afterwards some wondered aloud if she really was selectively mute. For her part Maria's mother would have liked to repeat this third step as she could hardly believe it, but there was no time to do that before the holidays began.

Maria went to France to see her grandmother and developed chicken-pox while she was there. This meant a late start for her as the new term had begun. We expected this to be another setback. Despite this, on return, she went eagerly to her new school and continued to speak to her class teacher and other staff, sometimes so volubly that they said that it was 'as though a tap had been turned on'. She was able to sing with the class and answer the register audibly, but would only speak to one other child. It seemed as though Maria was self-conscious about her accented English, felt more confident that adults would accept it, but feared that to the other children she would seem different.

We would have put into action a staged plan of fading other children one by one into situations where Maria spoke with her teacher and classroom helpers. However, as noted above, Maria's mother took the initiative at this point and continued to use stimulus fading techniques by inviting children home to play after school. Maria began to talk in school not only to children who had been to her home but to other children as well. Being able to talk confidently with other children acted as its own cumulative reinforcement. It was intrinsically satisfying and allowed her to perceive herself as socially competent. Thus Maria received both material and social reinforcement, and shaping and modelling were used in the course of our work with her. These behavioural techniques are often combined with stimulus fading.

Maria's assessment and treatment have been described in detail, because they illustrate several difficulties often experienced by practitioners, but not always described in the literature. There may be problems of coordination (and even of communication) when different agencies are involved with varying views about a child and an interest in different aspects of her welfare. This case also underlines the importance of ensuring that everyone involved has a clear understanding of the progress that has been made. Then, if unforeseen events interfere with plans for intervention, a plan can be revised quickly to build on progress to date while still being responsive to altered family or other needs. But, although this account illustrates a number of issues relating to the process of assessment, it does not show how that process can lay the basis for choosing a method of intervention in a wide variety of situations.

Basing the choice of intervention on behavioural assessment

The approach we recommend is based on the analysis of Labbe and Williamson (1984), whose review of a large number of behavioural case studies led them to develop a model for linking a strategy of intervention closely to the outcome of behavioural assessment. They suggested that there are five possible outcomes of the assessment of the child's speaking in what they called different 'test environments'. We have revised their table to introduce everyday language and to clarify the distinctions that are made between different 'assessment outcomes' (Table 7.4).

The crucial advantage of this approach is that it starts from a detailed analysis of the child's behaviour and situation. There is no presumption at the outset that any particular choice out of an eclectic selection of treatment strategies will be worth trying. The approach also takes account of the fact that the more complex treatment strategies will involve a greater number of steps. Therefore great care needs to be taken during assessment in order not to assume too readily that the outcome will demand, say, intervention strategy 5 when the simpler and more cost-effective strategy 2 would have been appropriate. Conversely, it is important not to miss out an essential step. For example, if a child speaks to only one or very few people in only one environment, new people will have to be faded in before fading of new settings.

It seems clear that, in some of the case studies on which Labbe and Williamson's review was based, less complex treatment plans could have been used, often with greater success, if an attempt had been made to link the planning of intervention more systematically with the results of the assessment. For example, in a report summarized in Chapter 4 Croghan and Craven (1982) described a treatment programme that lasted 2 years with an 8-year-old girl, JB. The programme was not succeeding after all this time, despite a combination of positive reinforcement, in vivo

Table 7.4 Linking intervention to the outcome of assessment

Level	Assessment outcome	Intervention strategy
1	Child speaks to most people in most settings but infrequently	The contingencies for speaking are changed in an appropriate environment, e.g. a new reward or reinforcer is introduced. Once the child is talking more normally in that environment, the reinforcer is faded. Speech is then maintained through natural reinforcement (i.e. the normal social rewards for speaking to others)
2	Child speaks to only one or a very few people in most settings	Stimulus fading of new people across key settings followed by contingency management as at level 1
3	Child speaks to most people in only one setting	Stimulus fading of new settings followed by contingency management as above
4	Child speaks to only one or a very few people in only one setting	Stimulus fading of new people and then of new settings, followed by contingency management as above
5	Child speaks to nobody able to help in the target setting	Response elicitation, then stimulus fading of people and settings, followed by contingency management as above

Adapted from Labbe and Williamson (1984).

desensitization, avoidance conditioning, modelling and the withdrawal of attention for not speaking. Rethinking the case helped the therapists to realize that the level of anxiety associated with speaking for JB had been underestimated. After systematic desensitization using a hierarchy of speech situations had been employed successfully, the therapists reviewed their case management and concluded that they had made a serious error in not considering stimulus fading. They had also made no attempt to include the mother in treatment, although this would have been possible. They noted that in fact there had been evidence from JB's history that this would have given good hope for success. The authors warn others against 'a premature commitment to particular behavioural strategies'.

A further analysis of the studies on which Labbe and Williamson based their argument initially suggested that there was little evidence for any cases with Outcome 3 (where the child speaks to most people in only one setting). The authors described the third outcome as unusual. They cited only one reference for it – Conrad, Delk and Williams (1974). That report seemed to us insufficiently detailed to justify differentiating it from Assessment Outcome 4, so we found it helpful to use a slightly simpler model that linked a smaller number of assessment outcomes with levels of intervention. We thought that this could be achieved without loss of information or accuracy. Subsequently we have encountered more examples of Assessment Outcome 3 and have reverted to Labbe and Williamson's tabulation (presented in Table 7.4).

Case studies to illustrate different levels of intervention

Outcome 1   *Speaks infrequently to most people in most settings*
Intervention level 1   Contingency management
If the child speaks only a little, perhaps in a very quiet voice or a whisper, there may be reason to intervene to improve frequency, volume or confidence in settings such as the classroom. These children are not best described as selectively mute, but they are anxious and lacking in social confidence. Some might become progressively more mute in certain circumstances. For example, if their reluctance to talk is because of the poor quality of their speech and they encounter teasing, they will be made to feel even more self-conscious and anxious. Children who present this risk are most often encountered in preschool provision and nurseries. Strategies learned from good practice in work with selectively mute children may be helpful. For instance, the member of staff with whom the child seems to be most comfortable may spend time with her, building up her confidence with one-to-one activities for short periods in the day. When she is talking more confidently other quiet children can be brought into this situation gradually, and contingency management may be used to help the child continue to speak frequently and at normal volume when that happens.

Most interventions linked to the problem of low frequency speech are planned and carried out at school, but Williamson et al. (1977b) described a programme with Kenneth (aged 7) who had been teased about his articulation difficulties. The intervention began in a clinic. They used a room with a one-way mirror so that Kenneth's mother could learn their methods and continue the programme at home. Baseline data were collected for responses to questions and spontaneous speech in the presence of different combinations of people. Tokens which could be 'cashed in' each day were used both at home and at school, and were accompanied with praise and attention. The frequency of Kenneth's replies to questions increased markedly, and there was some improvement in the frequency of spontaneous speech. Follow-up at home after 2 months and 1 year showed continued improvement.

Williamson et al. concluded that simple intervention procedures are sufficient and time saving when the children are not mute but speak 'reluctantly' in certain situations. They believed that a careful behavioural assessment will identify those children from whom a verbal response can occasionally be elicited. The main reason for using the minimum intervention that is effective is that it is less intrusive for the child, the family and the school. A second reason is that it will save costs. Williamson et al. estimated that in 1977 the use of less time-consuming procedures could save several hundred dollars per case. Presumably the figure is much higher now.

Outcome 2	*Child speaks to only one or a very few people in most settings*
Intervention level 2	**Stimulus fading of new people across key settings followed by contingency management**

Outcome 3	*Child speaks to most people in only one setting*
Intervention level 3	**Stimulus fading of new settings followed by contingency management**

In these situations the most effective intervention appears to be a stimulus fading strategy that extends the range of people to whom the child speaks across the range of settings felt to be important, e.g. school. The typical case of Outcome 2 is a child who will speak to her mother and siblings in several settings, but will stop speaking if anyone else appears. The typical case of Outcome 3 is a child who speaks to family and familiar visitors at home but to nobody in any other setting.

A good example of Outcome 2 was Sally (aged 6), a rather frail child, described by Reid et al. (1967). Sally would speak to no one but her immediate family, and not to them when a stranger was present. 'Just the sight of an outsider changed her manner from fluent activity to quiet preoccupation.' Sally had a long history of medical examinations because of a congenital heart defect. She tired quickly and had therefore spent a lot of time alone with her mother.

To help Sally the psychologists involved her mother in a marathon intervention in which at least three new people in turn were faded into the clinic playroom where she spoke with her mother. Stimulus fading was combined with reinforcement and took place over a whole day. The following week some of the steps were repeated, and after an initial hesitation Sally responded well to the introduction of more new people. During a third visit no reinforcement was used, and Sally's mother reported that she had begun to talk to people outside the home, e.g. at Sunday school. The therapists planned a continuing treatment programme in which Sally's talking was maintained by naturally occurring reinforcement, including peer group approval.

A similar clinic-based procedure was followed by Wulbert et al. (1973) with Emma (aged 6) and her mother. Again stimulus fading was combined with reinforcement, and finely graduated steps were used to fade in a sequence of different people. This study involved a careful research design. The workers alternated experimental periods when stimulus fading was used with control periods when it was not. They were able in this way to show that stimulus fading was a necessary part of the procedure. Other operant conditioning techniques were added if Emma did not respond to a request to speak. Again it was found that they were only effective if used in conjunction with stimulus control.

Because stimulus fading and reinforcement are often used together, the question arises – can positive reinforcement used alone be sufficient? Cunningham et al. (1983) reviewed the issue and could find only two studies where reinforcement alone had been used successfully with completely mute children. However, in both reports (Dmitriev and Hawkins, 1973; Piersel and Kratochwill, 1981) the authors appear to have achieved the difficult feat of ensuring that any non-verbal communication from the child was systematically ignored over an extended period of time. Moreover, it seems that reinforcement alone was tried ineffectively by a number of workers who went on to succeed with a combination of stimulus fading and reinforcement (Rasbury, 1974; Williamson et al., 1977b; Lipton, 1980). The reason for this appears to be that without a minimum level of speech in the target setting the children never obtain rewards for speaking, so that with positive reinforcement alone the reinforcement contingencies for speaking and non-speaking effectively do not change.

Cunningham et al. (1983) examined the converse: could stimulus fading be used effectively alone without reinforcement? John (aged 3) had a history of delayed expressive language. Both parents described themselves as having been shy children, and his father had not spoken to strangers until he was 4 or 5. In a preschool language group John would not speak to adults or children, although he spoke freely at home with his family. He was observed to speak with his mother in the preschool playroom, but stopped if a teacher entered. Family play sessions were set up in the playroom, and John's speech was established in that setting. John's teacher was gradually faded into the family play sessions, starting by remaining silently in a corner of the room, and then moving closer to John while he continued speaking. Once John spoke to her directly in the family session he continued to speak to her in other play settings into which another child was gradually introduced. The frequency of John's utterances per minute was recorded by videotaping sessions, which were then analysed. John's speech generalized to the classroom, and he was continuing to speak with peers and adults when followed up after 2 months and 6 months.

There are a number of cases in our own experience where stimulus fading alone has appeared to be swiftly effective. Presumably, however, natural social reinforcement is taking place concurrently, perhaps idiosyncratic to the child (e.g. through parents' expressions or tones of voice, possibly through increasing her own feelings of competence and thus relief from anxiety). As noted in Chapter 4, many of the workers who have used stimulus fading in school settings have focused on the child reading, sometimes aloud, and sometimes into a tape-recorder. Reading is often an activity which has been reinforced by parents over a period of time as a valued skill, and it may be an activity in which the child can sometimes feel more able than her peers.

In the case described by Afnan and Carr (1989), introduced in Chapter 4, the mother of Jenny (aged 6) devised a stimulus-fading programme on her own initiative which led to a stage when Jenny would read to her mother and teacher at school in the same room. Unfortunately, the next step was too abrupt. Without telling Jenny, her mother left the room where she was reading to the teacher and went home. Jenny clammed up and relapsed completely. Afnan and Carr re-introduced a stimulus-fading programme with token reinforcement that was to be delivered by Jenny's father in the evening. In each reading session at school the distance between Jenny and her mother was to be gradually increased, and that between Jenny and her teacher decreased. Importantly, the steps in the programme were to be decided by the mother, but Jenny was to have control over the timing of their introduction and was to be told that the failure of the previous attempt was because she had not been 'ready' for the next step. This 'reframing' seems to have taken the pressure off Jenny and her mother, because the day after the plan had been explained to her Jenny whispered to her mother in school, and her mother followed this lead by reinforcing her for spontaneous speech in school. Of her own accord, Jenny began to increase the number of people with whom she spoke. An important element of the intervention was parallel work on communication and attitudes within the family, but this could not have been successful on its own without the stimulus-fading strategy.

Stimulus fading can be carried out in school with anyone with whom speaking has been established. It does not need to be a parent. In a study described in Chapter 4 Rosenbaum and Kellman (1973) used stimulus fading in school with a 9-year-old girl who had not spoken in class for 2 years. The key figure was a speech therapist, who had established speech in a one-to-one setting with reinforcement, and then transferred speaking to the girl's classroom, using successive approximations.

Scott (1977) working with Linda, a very shy 6-year-old, made good use of a routine already established at school, whereby Linda did her reading into a tape-recorder alone in a quiet room in school. The psychologist knew Linda quite well, as she had attended a play therapy group in the clinic for 6 months where she had become more relaxed though she never spoke or participated. Linda was now about to move to a new school, and she and her mother were feeling very anxious about it. The intervention involved gradually introducing Scott into a room in the clinic where Linda read into a tape-recorder answers to written questions about a picture. There were six stages through which Scott moved from outside the room and out of view steadily closer until she was sitting face to face with Linda at the same table. The criterion for each move was that Linda had given 10 consecutive appropriate responses with Scott in the previous position. At this stage the written questions were removed, and Linda answered similar questions previously taped by Scott, still recording her responses. Then the tape-recorder was taken away, and Linda replied to verbal questions from Scott. After she had successfully met the criterion in that condition, the setting was moved to another room and then a game of 'I spy' was introduced in which Linda first had to reply to questions with 'yes' or no' and then had to ask the questions.

At this stage a series of different adults, including her past and present teacher and two adults not met before, were introduced as observers into the session, listening to the first 10 questions, taking over the questioning for the next 10 in Scott's presence, and then asking another 10 while Scott was out of the room. Following this, the new adult took Linda into the playroom to join Scott for a game of 'I spy'. At last the programme was transferred to Linda's classroom with her teacher, with the intention of starting from an empty classroom and gradually increasing the proximity of other children. There was an initial setback when Linda did not respond if there was another child present, whatever the distance between them. This was overcome by reintroducing Scott for a session in the library corner of the classroom where Scott repeated the former routine with Linda and then introduced six children from Linda's group one by one until Linda was responding in a group of seven children. The same process was repeated with the children in the main part of the classroom, first by Scott and then by the class teacher.

This report has been quoted at length, because it used a response that was already in the child's repertoire and gradually increased not only the closeness of the therapist but the level of response required. (This is often called the **changing criterion design** – see Chapter 9.) Although it would seem that the intervention could have been completed more quickly if it had taken place in Linda's school from the beginning, the total length of the programme was only 4 weeks. It is a good example of how desensitization may sometimes be used to bring a child to the point where stimulus fading can be the vehicle for generalization across new people and new situations.

Outcome 4	*Child speaks to only one or very few people in only one setting*
Intervention level 4	**Stimulus fading of new people and then of new settings, followed by contingency management**

When a child speaks to one or a very few people in only one setting (e.g. home) but to nobody in another key setting (e.g. school), new people and settings must both be faded in. The aim of the first stage is that the child should be helped to speak to a new person in the home setting. Then a new aim is set – that the child should speak to that person in the target setting. After that, there will be generalization to other people in the target setting.

If on the behavioural assessment the child appears to talk to only one or two people, perhaps only the immediate family in the home, intervention will have to start in that setting. The first stage of stimulus fading will be to fade in new people and then to fade in new settings. It will be necessary to start by gradually introducing another person into the home, with the aim that, as the child becomes accustomed to that person, she will speak to her mother in that person's presence. As the stimulus control for speaking becomes transferred she will begin to speak to that person both with and without her mother present. That may take several visits.

There are strong arguments for work with very young selectively mute children to be carried out in their homes, at least initially. Tessa was referred to a child guidance clinic at the age of 4 years 11 months because she had become totally mute, even at home, communicating solely by gesture. This development occurred after an illness when it had been necessary for her to see a doctor, despite her fear of strangers. Sluckin and Jehu (1969) described her early history. According to her parents, Tessa had always been a stubborn child (e.g. over mealtimes and toilet training), but her development had been normal. However, around the age of 4, she suddenly became rather shy and spoke to only a limited number of people.

When Sluckin visited the family a few days after Tessa had been referred, she found that she had begun to talk again to her family, but remained mute with others, even in the home. Sluckin felt that Tessa's mother was reinforcing her mutism and suggested rewarding more appropriate behaviour. Within the next few months Tessa started school, and although she settled well, did not speak to other children or to teachers.In her second term concern increased. Sluckin noted that although Tessa seemed to enjoy communicating with her in 'a rather flirtatious way', she would not speak to her, or to her mother in Sluckin's presence.

After further discussion with Tessa's mother, Sluckin proposed that she would reward Tessa with a sweet if she would read to her mother while she (Sluckin) was there. Whispering just a line was rewarded at first, and then more was asked, both in amount and audibility, while at the same time Sluckin gradually increased her proximity to Tessa. By the end of 8 weeks, Tessa was reading and talking to her mother in loud whispers, while Sluckin sat next to them on the settee. Sluckin then suggested taping Tessa, and a series of songs and conversations were recorded and played back by Tessa to Sluckin and finally to her headteacher at school. Tessa's mother then began to visit the school regularly, and with her, Tessa would sometimes (but not always) read to the headteacher.

Following this, Sluckin promised Tessa stars for reading, and while she was reading and enthusiastically collecting stars, her mother left the room and Tessa continued to read. After several similar sessions, Tessa began to talk to Sluckin, even in the mother's absence. Shortly after this she began to talk to the headteacher at school. Progress was maintained after the summer holidays, and Tessa began to speak spontaneously to most people. (A similar programme with another child is described by Sluckin, 1977.)

Conrad, Delk and Williams (1974) offer a good illustration of the need for a two-stage programme, first introducing a new stimulus person into the home, and then, when speech is established with that person, transferring to new settings. A Native American Indian girl who had never spoken in school was able to speak to a member of the professional team from the same cultural group when he was faded into her home setting. Once she was speaking to him with and without her mother present, this was transferred to another setting, the clinic, and again new people were carefully faded into the clinic setting, including a friend from school and the class teacher. This was done using activities chosen to create a school-like atmosphere. Finally, similar sessions were held at school, first with a small group of five children, and then with the whole class. This case underlines the value, where a child comes from a cultural or linguistic minority, of involving an adult from the same community at an early stage in stimulus fading. The opportunity of doing this was fortunately available in the case of Maria (see above). The contribution of Lily in that case undoubtedly accelerated the pace of the intervention.

Richards and Hansen (1978) provide another example of a carefully staged procedure (see Chapter 4). Both they and Rasbury (1974) used stimulus fading on the route to school with a progressively higher criterion.

Outcome 5	*Child speaks to nobody who is available to help in the target setting*
Intervention level 5	**Response elicitation, then stimulus fading of people and settings, followed by contingency management**

The first stage of intervention at this level can be described under the general heading of **response elicitation** – trying to initiate speech through different 'packages' of operant techniques. From case studies it is clear that this level of intervention will not be sufficient on its own. Further work at levels 2, 3 or 4 (stimulus fading) and then also at level 1 (contingency management) will be necessary before the process is complete. It will therefore take considerably longer to carry out, and there are other disadvantages too. These approaches are usually school-based because that is the target setting. They are sometimes adopted in residential settings for the same reason. It is advisable to explore thoroughly at the outset whether any obstacles to a stimulus-fading programme can be overcome before accepting that a level 5 intervention is necessary. Intervention at levels 2, 3 or 4 is less intrusive for the child, more economic in terms of time, and probably likely to have a higher chance of success. However, in the published reports of level 5 interventions there is seldom any detailed account of whether such an approach was considered or whether any attempt was made to enlist the parents' help. There are many reasons why parents may be unable to help. For example, they may be ill or have other pressures on their time, or they may be unsure and unconfident about their ability to work with the teachers in school.

There are several approaches which should be considered before beginning a level 5 intervention. First, when applying Labbe and Williamson's framework, even if it appears that there is 'nobody available to help in the target setting', it is often possible to find someone who will be willing to visit the home to establish speech with the child and mother in that setting and then follow a stimulus-fading procedure. Much progress can be made in this way, as was shown in the study by Conrad and his colleagues quoted above. It needs to be someone who can be accepted both by the family and by the school where the later stages of the programme will be carried out.

When the parents or others with whom the child is able to talk are not available or not able to take part in a stimulus-fading programme in the target setting, it has often been necessary to elicit speech with a new person in a safe setting in order to reach the basis for intervention strategy levels 3 or 4. A relatively straightforward example was given by Clayton (1981) working in school with Clarissa (aged 6) who had not spoken at playgroup or school over a period of 3 years. A further problem was that she screamed for an hour each morning before coming to school. Clayton's intervention began in a small room near the classroom with the door shut where he elicited speech using social and token reinforcement. After 4–5 sessions the class teacher and Clarissa's two closest friends were faded in. Reading aloud to the class teacher was selected as the next task. It was to be tackled as a group and rewarded by stickers. Once this was achieved in the side room, the group repeated it first in the empty classroom and then with the whole class present. At the next stage, during the reading sessions, Clarissa was sent to take messages around the school. If any were inaudible she had to return to the classroom, practise and try again. Follow-up 9 months later showed that the new behaviour had been maintained and that Clarissa now spoke spontaneously to other children and to teachers. Her parents reported that she no longer screamed in the mornings.

However, it may not be possible for psychologists to allocate so much time to work with a selectively mute child at school themselves. The manual by Johnson and Wintgens (2001) gives many suggestions to enable a key worker such as a learning support assistant to elicit responses through a variety of games and other activities. They recommend support for the key worker from a speech and language therapist or psychologist who has worked with similar children in the past. They use some of the level 5 techniques such as shaping, but point out that stimulus fading (which they describe as 'sliding in') and positive reinforcement will also be needed to complete the process.

Usually level 5 interventions involve greater challenges at the first stage when the child's anxiety is particularly high. Eliciting speech to a new stimulus figure in a setting where speech is not established typically proves very difficult. Another reason for not attempting interventions at this level is that once an attempt has failed the child's resistance to attempts in this setting is often increased. Some of the techniques which have already been described in combination with earlier levels of intervention, especially shaping, modelling and reinforcement, can also be used to elicit speech. In some cases aversive techniques have been used for this purpose, e.g. response cost, overcorrection, time out and escape/avoidance. Each of these will be described briefly, although overcorrection, time out and escape/avoidance may be seen by the child as punitive and are best avoided.

Shaping

This technique is often used in teaching children with severe learning difficulties and has been applied to training skills in other areas of behaviour and development. It involves analysing the target skill and breaking it down into component steps, one of which is already in the child's repertoire. That step can be easily elicited and reinforced. Then the therapist restricts reinforcement to those responses which approximate most closely to the next steps in the sequence. Physical prompts and auditory or visual cues are often used to speed up the initial stages and are faded out when no longer needed. In a severe case shaping communication skills with a selectively mute child might move through a lengthy series of steps towards full communication. The exact sequence will vary according to what the child finds easy and difficult. In the case of Amy (aged 7) treated by Austad, Sininger and Stricken (1980) the sequence was – 'opening mouth as though yawning, making simple sounds with mouth open, verbalizing vowel sounds, verbalizing consonant sounds, verbalizing parts of specific words, verbalizing one half of her own name, verbalizing her full name, repeating what therapist said, answering questions with one word, answering questions with more than one word, answering questions with sentences, spontaneously generating sentences in a ten-minute period, and increasing the loudness of speech'.

Modelling

One of the targets for which shaping is used may be to help the child to imitate actions or sounds. Modelling is often combined with shaping: the target response is modelled, the child's response is prompted and then reinforced. To begin with, it may be necessary to have a third person to model the target response. It should be noted that the personal qualities of the model may have a strong effect on the child's willingness to imitate the actions (Bozigar and Hansen, 1984; Winter, 1984). With selectively mute children the familiarity of the model may be an important factor – and may indeed perhaps be operating covertly in the early stages of stimulus fading carried out at home. (Self-modelling, which is a different process, was described in Chapter 4.)

Cunningham et al. (1983) described an intervention that exemplifies the way in which modelling and shaping may lay the basis for work at levels 1–4. Steven (aged 15) had not spoken at school since he was 5, but communicated with teachers and children in gestures and writing. 'After many unsuccessful intervention attempts by school personnel' he was referred to an adolescent psychiatric clinic at John Hopkins University, Baltimore and then transferred to an inpatient unit in the Kennedy Institute for Handicapped Children. He again refused to speak, but responded with gestures and written answers. Shaping with modelling was used in the first of four phases of treatment. He progressed through imitating motor responses, facial gestures and sounds to mouthing and finally whispering answers to questions. The second phase involved stimulus fading of both people and settings. The third phase initiated generalization by reinforced practice procedures. (Steven carried a card and collected the signatures of people to whom he spoke.) A fourth phase was needed to establish normal conversational volume through prompting, fading and successive approximation procedures, followed by token reinforcement. On follow-up by telephone 1 and 2 months after treatment Steven's parents said he spoke consistently at school and to other children. The first step towards this had required response elicitation in the unpromising circumstances of an inpatient stay after 10 years' selective silence.

Reinforcement sampling

Sometimes non-contingent reinforcement (reinforcement that is not linked to the target response) is given in the first session of response elicitation to show the child that reinforcement is available to her. Otherwise, if the target response (even the first target in a shaping sequence) is rare in the child's behaviour, she may never experience the reinforcement at all. Reinforcement sampling may sometimes start with the person modelling the target response being reinforced. Another strategy described in several reports on selective mutism is that the child is allowed a 'taster'. This overcomes the difficulty of using positive reinforcement with a child who does not speak at all in some settings. For example, Austad, Sininger and Stricken (1980) allowed Amy to play with a pet rabbit so that the reward for speaking could be anticipated and its reinforcement value increased. The ultimate goal of her programme was set as earning the right to take this rabbit home as her own pet.

Similarly, Williamson et al. (1977b) allowed Crissy (aged 7) limited time to 'sample' the reward of roller skates. This technique was used after shaping alone had failed to get Crissy to imitate a sound, and followed sessions using Crissy's mother to model words, combined with stimulus fading in which the therapist gradually increased his proximity to Crissy and her mother. The use of the skates for 3 days was contingent on responding to the therapist in the room, and complete ownership was gained after she had read to her class for 10 minutes.

Like shaping and modelling, reinforcement sampling attempts to elicit speech through positive reinforcement alone, but can be used in combination with other strategies. The remaining items in the list of strategies involve forms of negative reinforcement. These include increasing the probability of target behaviour occurring by the removal of unpleasant consequences (e.g. escape/avoidance) or decreasing unwanted behaviour such as non-speaking either by removing pleasant consequences (e.g. response cost and time out) or by applying unpleasant consequences (e.g. overcorrection). All these procedures can be seen as aversive, although theoretically only overcorrection is punishment.

Response cost

If the child fails to speak, she loses opportunities for reinforcement. This technique has featured in a number of studies, most often when tokens are used for positive reinforcement. It works well in situations where the child values the rewards. Griffith et al. (1975) describe how response cost through loss of points for not speaking to peers was used with a 6-year-old boy in one class setting to maintain the value of the points system because he was earning too many in another class setting (his reading group). The use of the response cost procedure coincided with an increase in spontaneous speech to peers. Follow-up 3 months later showed continued improvement (see also Sanok and Striefel, 1979).

Overcorrection

Overcorrection in the sense of positive practice was used by Matson et al. (1979) with Todd (aged 9) who had not spoken for 3 years. Despite this, until recently he had made normal progress in school. Intervention took place in a room on a ward in the hospital for emotionally disturbed children where Todd was an inpatient. In baseline sessions Todd was asked to name picture cards and answer questions with yes or no. Similar cards were used in treatment sessions, but in addition the therapist modelled the response for Todd after showing him the card. For each correct response Todd was praised and given a penny and a paper slip entitling him to a certain amount of free time. If he did not answer correctly he had to write out 10 times the word he should have imitated. This combined intervention 'package' of modelling, reinforcement and overcorrection elicited responses from Todd, but the effect was highly stimulus specific and did not generalize to two other therapists introduced later into the sessions. However, on the ward, Todd began to say words that had not been trained in the intervention phase, and he was continuing to do this 4 months after the study began.

Time out

The proper use of this procedure makes it clear that it is time out from positive reinforcement. It marks out a short time when, following undesired behaviour, the opportunity of earning rewards is removed. It was used in combination with positive reinforcement and stimulus fading by Wulbert et al. (1973). There are very few instances of time out being used with selectively mute children, as it could reasonably be expected to increase anxiety. Because time out should have a predetermined time limit set in advance, it is not equivalent to the periods of being isolated or ignored that feature in some of the escape/avoidance procedures to be discussed next.

Escape/avoidance

In these procedures the child is released from the aversive situation when she makes the required response. In most of the reports which describe these procedures as an intervention to increase speaking, the child is required to say one word before being allowed to leave the classroom or the clinic. Sometimes this is at the end of the day, when the child is prevented from going home (e.g. Halpern, Hammond and Cohen, 1971). Williamson et al. (1977b) described an escape procedure which was used with Michael (aged 8) to produce a one-word response when shaping and modelling had not succeeded. Michael was told he would receive a dollar and be able to leave the clinic for a rest break with his mother if he said 'home'. If he did not respond he would be left alone in the room for 20 minutes and then he would again be asked to respond. This combined positive and negative reinforcement is a powerful intervention package and had the desired result: he increased his rate of responding from zero previously to 40% in the first session and 100% in the fourth session.

The opportunity to escape may sometimes be sufficient reinforcement in itself: An example of what the authors termed a 'mild aversive' being used as part of a systematic intervention was described by Watson and Kramer (1992) who arranged for a child to be kept in during break-time if he did not achieve his daily speaking target in the classroom. A similar approach was employed by Lumb and Wolff (1988) who described their work with Jackie, an able 11-year-old who had acquired a number of privileges because of her status as a non-speaker. Her parents and teachers agreed that it was important for her to start to speak in her final year at primary school before she transferred to secondary school. It was explained to her that all privileges would be removed and restored only as a reward for talking. She was not allowed to sit with her friends in class or to go out to play, and had to eat lunch alone. After initial anger and sulks on the first day Jackie began to reply with one-word answers on the second day, and gradually increased the length and quality of her answers until she was asking and responding, though not spontaneously initiating conversation. Follow-up after transfer to her new school showed that she was now talking normally.

A similar approach has frequently been reported by teachers to one of the authors (SB), usually only when it has been successful. This was often undertaken on their own initiative, typically when there was no access to external advice. However, a number of children have been referred after at least one such attempt has failed. Susie, who was then 6, had forgotten her bus fare. She let the school bus depart without her, remaining obstinately silent as she wept, refusing to say 'please' to her teacher who had offered the money to her if she spoke. Her teacher then had to drive the child home and explain to her parents what had happened. Using these approaches is not recommended, especially if they are undertaken in isolation and not as part of a carefully planned sequence of intervention.

Other more extreme examples of the use of escape/avoidance procedures can be found in Shaw (1971) and Van der Kooy and Webster (1975), but are not described here in detail. They both deal with aversive uses of avoidance procedures with children in residential settings and are of theoretical interest only. A wide range of positive methods is available. The use of extreme negative approaches seems unnecessary as well as ethically dubious.

A much more cautious approach to the use of escape/avoidance procedures was adopted by Lysne (1995). He argued that they should not be used with young children and should never be the first method tried. He also felt that before these approaches were used, the therapists should have persuasive indications that a positive outcome was likely. He stressed the importance of 'creating a trustful relationship' between the implementing person and the child. Lysne worked with a 14-year-old boy who had become reluctant to speak outside the home when he was 4 and did not speak there if visitors came, becoming angry if he spoke accidentally. He had had a significant and upsetting early separation when admitted to hospital as a baby.

His early speech and language development had seemed normal. He was the youngest of three boys, and his mother was thought to be overprotective of him. She did not warn the school about his difficulties until just before he started at the age of 7. He was referred for help in his first year and seen by a psychologist and a speech and language therapist. During the next 2 years he attended a local child psychiatric clinic. Later Lysne tried a variety of behavioural approaches, including stimulus fading and reinforcement sampling, but without result. Finally it was decided to try an escape procedure after extensive assessment of how he was likely to react to this. His parents and others concerned with his care agreed that it might help him to overcome his barriers and probably would not do him any harm.

This intervention was presented to him as a training programme based on an 'agreement ' between the boy and Lysne. For the first two sessions he had to imitate animal noises, which he did reluctantly. In the third session he had to say one word to be released and this was difficult for both of them. He tried to 'press out some sounds' which were not acceptable but finally managed to say 'yes' to a question. He and Lysne rewarded themselves with chocolate. This was a breakthrough, and he then made rapid progress. Later he was able to talk about his mutism: 'He knew each time he left home that he would not speak . . . but he did watch out when provoked by someone to speak'. This has been quoted at length, because it is so clear that Lysne's cautious approach and evident care for the boy's well-being established a relationship of trust. That was what made the escape/avoidance procedure ethically acceptable and was part of the basis of its success. Subsequently new people and settings in school were faded in with reinforcement, followed by generalization.

A case study illustrating the value of behavioural assessment and its limitations

Michael, who was nearly 8, had not spoken at playgroup, in the nursery class or in his first years at school. There was great concern about his progress with school work, and his mother had been unsuccessful in seeking help for his speech and language difficulties (which included a problem of articulation). The therapist was unable to see him at home, and he would not speak to her in the clinic.

The school was in special measures after an inspection, and the teachers' morale was low. A large number of children with learning and behavioural difficulties were waiting for assessment. The headteacher did not encourage the idea of home visits by staff because he felt they were under too much pressure. Because of the school's difficulties it had been allocated six visits from the educational psychologist over one term. It was agreed that the psychologist would visit Michael and his family at home in the evening after each visit to the school.

When Michael's mother met her at school, she was pleased with the idea of a home visit. She commented: 'He'll talk to anyone at school when he's got to know them'. She still blamed herself for leaving Michael at playgroup when he was 2 because it had been suggested that that would help his speech. 'I could hear his screaming all the way down the road.' She remembered that she and her sisters had all been very shy at school.

Both she and Michael were anxious when the psychologist arrived, but he warmed up when his mother talked about their recent day out at a local theme park. He rushed upstairs and found a map and pointed out the best rides, highlighting the one where his Dad had felt sick. Endearingly, he gave the psychologist his spare copy of the map so that she would know which were the best rides. On the next visit he was more confident, partly because of competition from his younger sister who wanted her share of attention as she had been at a friend's house on the previous occasion. The children's routine included reading tasks sent home by the school. They both struggled with books that made demands well below the level that might have been expected for their age. Michael had poor articulation and also experienced difficulties with pencil control. He would eventually require extra help based on a full assessment of his special educational needs, but there was never any doubt that helping him to speak in school was the first priority. Because of the situation at the school it was not possible to bring any of the staff into the setting where he spoke comfortably, at home, so the next stage was to explore his ability to speak in a third setting.

On the next visit Michael, his mother and sister walked round the housing estate with the psychologist. He continued to talk and waved to some of the boys playing football who shouted back in a friendly way. He also spoke to his mother in the supermarket, but only in a very quiet voice. She was pleased with his progress but felt school would be the real barrier. With the agreement of the headteacher the next visit took place in his classroom about 2 hours after school had finished. There were cleaners and one or two teachers around, but this did not prevent Michael talking with his sister as they chalked on the blackboard and giggled. This was repeated the following week. Because this visit had gone well it was arranged that the class teacher would join them the following week. Both Michael and the teacher were uneasy. He was willing to play the card game 'Snap', but often held back a verbal response, losing opportunities to win at the game. When sweets were introduced as rewards for winning each round he was able to answer 'snap', but there was none of the spontaneous speech he had produced at home and on the previous visit to school. This was repeated in another visit after school, but it was clear that several more steps would be needed before Michael would be able to talk with his teachers in school.

With agreement from the school and the family Michael and the psychologist worked in the special needs room for a session after school on games which he had brought from home. In this situation he spoke quite freely, but when it was repeated during the school day, he was unable to speak at all. He looked at the psychologist apologetically and went very red. She had not initially appreciated the implications of the large glass panel in the door to the corridor through which he could see people passing and knew they could see him. She said that she had made a mistake: using the room in school time was too difficult at the moment, and she would find another one. The special educational needs coordinator

(SENCO) suggested a little room behind the dining hall which was always empty after lunch. Michael liked this place, which he had never been allowed into before. He read to the psychologist there from his reading book with some support. He agreed he could do this with one of the learning support assistants (LSA), and this was accomplished immediately on the same day with the reward of a gold point from the SENCO and a note to take home telling his mother how well he had done.

It is essential that a school takes steps to ensure that a child generalizes their new-found ability to speak there. It is sometimes assumed that progress will be automatic once a child has spoken to an LSA or the class teacher. Michael's next teacher carefully built on the progress that had been made by steadily expanding the range of contacts and extending the size of the groups in which he was called upon to talk, so he made good progress throughout his year with her. After a formal assessment of his special educational needs, provision was made for speech and language therapy in school and to give him additional support in class.

He was followed up subsequently for 3 years. During that period he continued to make progress. At the time of the last enquiry he was speaking in most school settings but seldom asked questions himself spontaneously. He still had difficulties with literacy skills and in other areas of the curriculum, which upset him at times. He was much more confident and had recently insisted on going with his class on a week-long school trip, even though his parents and teachers had been very anxious about it and he needed to take medication for nocturnal enuresis while away. The teachers and assistants on the trip were proud of him because he coped so well. He took part in all activities, including abseiling and caving, and worked well with a partner. Shortly after this, during a 'hobbies week' at the end of the summer term, he showed that he had a real talent for gardening and could help other children with their plots – an unusual role for a boy who fell behind his age peers in most school activities.

The intervention to help Michael was based on an assessment of his patterns of speech across several different settings and of the contingencies affecting his communication in the target setting. At the beginning of the intervention he was assessed at level 3 – talking to most people at home, to a number of people around the estate where he lived and to nobody at all at school. Ideally, following the model derived from Labbe and Williamson (1984), the psychologist would have faded one or more people from the target setting (teachers) into the setting where he was speaking freely (home). An evaluation of ecological factors made it clear that that was not possible. So the intervention began at level 4 – fading his sister and mother and then the psychologist into the school setting, modifying that setting by using it when other pupils and staff were not present. But the intervention did not proceed as smoothly as it could have done, because the assessment did not analyse in sufficient detail some of the contingencies influencing Michael's speech. He experienced the same setting very differently at different times. Fear of being observed by others and feeling acutely embarrassed when unable to meet a demand were both important factors in his difficulties and might have been taken into account earlier if the assessment had covered such issues. In the next section we discuss recent developments in analogue assessment and functional analysis. If a strategy incorporating these elements had been implemented with Michael, he might have made quicker progress.

The value of functional analysis

There are factors in a child's social environment which may maintain non-speaking and which are not adequately covered in the grids that we presented earlier or in the assessment strategy that we have described. Sanok and Ascione (1979) examined some of the methodological issues that arose from the early accounts of behavioural treatment. They maintained that few accounts of behavioural intervention had demonstrated effectiveness in producing a comprehensive change in speaking habits (for example, in spontaneous as well as prompted speech) or an improvement across different settings. They suggested a number of reasons for this. The first was that working towards generalization was not incorporated in treatment plans. The second reason was that, because it was so difficult, few workers tried to 're-programme' those around the child who were reinforcing inappropriate non-verbal responses. Fundamental to these problems was the lack of a sufficiently rigorous behavioural assessment. As they saw it, this needed to include a functional analysis of the exact antecedent conditions which failed to produce verbal responses or produced inadequate responses such as whispering. They argued that functional analysis would be extremely useful in identifying the factors which maintain mutism and ways of altering them to facilitate normal speech communication. At the time their initiative was not followed up in a systematic way, though some researchers and clinicians took the main principle on board.

When Schill, Kratochwill and Gardner (1996a) reported on their later investigations of strategies of systematic functional analysis of selective mutism, they drew upon work in their department by Twernbold (1996). He had examined the efficacy of a model of functional analysis to analyse the demand conditions affecting the restricted speech of a 4-year-old boy who had some articulation problems. The assessment was in two parts. During the first phase the parents were interviewed using a simple checklist, the Functional Diagnostic Profile, in order to record systematically their description of their son and their account of the people and settings where he spoke or was silent. On that basis hypotheses were formed about the demand conditions that might facilitate or inhibit the child's speech. During the second phase a more rigorous 'analogue assessment' technique was employed. In this strategy the aim was to replicate in the clinic some of the conditions that were encountered in the child's daily experience elsewhere. The conditions were varied systematically so as to identify more precisely the demand conditions that facilitated or inhibited speech. Thus during the analogue assessment the psychologist conducted a series of what were, in effect, mini-experiments to confirm or invalidate the hypotheses that had been developed on the basis of descriptive accounts by those close to the child.

During the assessment it emerged that:

- The child spoke more frequently in an unstructured free-play setting than in a structured setting in which he was faced with specific demands for speech.
- He spoke more frequently when interacting freely with his father than when with his mother or with an unfamiliar adult.
- His father tended to join in play activities with him and to allow him to lead them, whereas his mother spoke more herself when they were together and took more of a lead both in the play and in the conversation. When his mother posed a question, she was more likely to answer it herself after a pause, thus allowing him to avoid the need to answer it. His father was less likely to do that, and also reacted in a different way when he did speak, regularly repeating his words as though to confirm what he had said.

Thus functional analysis helped the psychologist to develop hypotheses about the environmental and personal factors that might maintain the child's mutism across different settings. On the basis of the observations and the hypotheses built from them the psychologist developed a series of recommendations for how parents, teachers and other adults should interact with the child in order to encourage him to extend his speaking habits beyond the restricted settings in which he was then speaking:

- Structure play times loosely, allowing him to direct the course of play and joining in with him, so that he feels comfortable with an adult present.
- Phrase questions as open-ended statements which he can complete rather than giving him specific directives to talk.
- Use modelling techniques when he fails to give a verbal response to a question rather than allowing him to escape the demand.
- When he speaks, repeat what he says so as to confirm that he has been understood.

There are many advantages to conducting such assessments, where possible, in the natural settings in which the child's behaviour occurs – the home and the school. The video and audio recordings that were made in Twernbold's case study could now be undertaken in a child's home as the equipment is more readily available and is very easy to set up. As we indicated earlier, we see functional assessment as complementing Labbe and Williamson's framework in a very useful way. An informal interview with parents and teachers may suggest some of the factors that maintain the child's mutism. An analogue assessment using recording techniques can then allow the parents and professionals in regular contact with the child to see and hear for themselves how changing the conditions they create for speaking could be beneficial. In a later study Schill, Kratochwill and Gardner (1996b) employed the same approach in work with an 8-year-old girl but, instead of carrying out all the assessment at the clinic, taught the analogue assessment techniques to her parents so that they could conduct the assessment themselves at home. At the same time a teacher was involved with the parents in carrying out replication procedures at school.

An earlier study from the same department illustrates the potential advantages of combining functional analysis with behavioural assessment employing the Labbe and Williamson model. Sheridan, Kratochwill and Ramirez (1995) had argued that assessment should provide information to help in the planning of intervention. Their subject was Stacy, a child who had been adopted at the age of 3. When she was about 3 she was involved in a boating accident with her adoptive father, who died. At that time she developed nocturnal enuresis, which persisted. When she was referred she was 6, and had not spoken in any school setting since starting preschool three years earlier.

Their assessment had three aims – to complete a formal diagnosis demonstrating that Stacy was selectively mute within the current DSM classification, to carry out a functional analysis of her mute behaviour and to evaluate the effects of the intervention. The conditions surrounding her behaviour were to be analysed, and further hypotheses developed into a plan of intervention. Indirect measures (structured interviews, questionnaires and checklists) and direct measures (observations, tape recordings, functional assessment and Matson's fear thermometer) were included. Data were collected in a university clinic, at Stacy's home and at her school. Audiotapes of her speech at home were collected, and her mother completed records of her speech in specific situations.

Analogue assessments were carried out in the clinic, using a one-way mirror and audio and video recording. Analysis showed that when Stacy did not answer a direct question her mother or other people often 'helped' by answering for her. The situations where Stacy was expected to answer and did not were also replicated with questions of the kind that allowed a gesture or a yes/no response. Others, especially children, often answered for her, and nobody seemed to expect a verbal response. Her mother said that Stacy's main difficulty was speaking to adults at school. She also said that Stacy had sometimes spoken to her at school and to a school bus driver, though it appears that unfortunately this was not recorded. After consultation and reference to Labbe and Williamson's model, it was decided that, as Stacy was not speaking to any available person in the school setting, the team would employ a response elicitation intervention at school with modelling, shaping and positive reinforcement. Other strategies were used to change the behaviour of those around her: peer prompting from a child whom she knew well, asking other children not to answer for her and encouraging teachers to phrase questions so that she could not respond with gestures.

These strategies were tried for 5 months without effect; in fact, Stacy showed 'extreme resistance' to them. At a review meeting a further analysis was made using the Labbe and Williamson model. It was decided that, as she spoke to her mother in some settings, an attempt could be made to transfer this to school, and a 'Secret Message' game was set up using stimulus fading and positive reinforcement, involving first her teacher and then her peers. The settings changed over four phases. Initially they worked in the staffroom, where Stacy had no difficulty in speaking to her mother. They created an audiotape of a message that Stacy had written earlier. This was repeated in the library, which was closer to the classroom. Her teacher was gradually brought in, moving stage by stage closer to the table where they sat. As the demands increased Stacy found it increasingly difficult but still co-operated enough to gain reinforcement. However, her progress halted when she was asked to read the message aloud to her teacher when she was sitting facing her. She refused at this point and was upset. But, once the task was broken down into smaller steps, at first requiring no eye contact, she was able to make further progress, and within days was able to speak to her mother and the teacher together.

In the next phase the programme was moved into the classroom. It began with a new child who had just started at the school (and to whom Stacy had never been unable to speak). Initially she whispered to her when other children were present and spoke aloud to her when they were alone. Other children were faded in gradually in each session, and then Stacy spoke in small group situations. In all this process took 31 days – a significant contrast to the 5 months of unsuccessful work employing the first approach. Unfortunately at this point term ended before generalization could be established to other settings and children.

An analysis of this case study reinforces the case for ensuring that opportunities are taken to use simple strategies of intervention with people and settings where a child speaks confidently. It is important that these are not overlooked in favour of more complicated plans. We have found, working in schools, that assessment outcome 3 in the Labbe and Williamson model, 'Child speaks to nobody available to help in the target setting', is often understood as – 'Child speaks to nobody **immediately** available to help . . .' and thus mistakenly excludes the possibility of 'someone **becoming available** to help in the target setting'. We suggest that the description of level 3 assessment and intervention should be rephrased as a question 'Is there anyone to whom the child speaks who could be available to help in school or nursery?' If an intervention using response elicitation fails it can often make the situation more damaging for the child and parents and sometimes impair relationships.

A staged procedure for assessment and intervention

The outline of a staged procedure for assessment and intervention can now be summarized. Readers familiar with the version introduced in the first edition of this text will see that we have now revised it to take account of developments in the use of functional analysis with selectively mute children.

1. Determine whether a primary focus on selective mutism is justified by checking whether any other aspects of the child's behaviour are causing serious concern to the parents or others. In some cases these may, in fact, be related to the selective use of speech.
2. Obtain systematic, descriptive information on the child's speech and non-verbal communication in a wide variety of settings and with different people. This should include whether the child's silence in a target setting is being reinforced in any way by how other people respond to them.
3. At this point, the outcome of the behavioural assessment should clearly indicate the required level of intervention within the Labbe and Williamson framework. Discuss this with the parents and those involved with the child in the target settings. It is important that everyone who will be involved in carrying out the intervention has an opportunity for questions and discussion. Agree together the best way of explaining the intervention to the child.
4. On the basis of the descriptive behavioural assessment hypotheses will have been developed about the contingencies or demand conditions that may facilitate or inhibit the child's speech. Where there are any contradictions or significant gaps in the information obtained, a further functional analysis will be required, and parents or teachers may be asked to participate in mini-experiments as part of an analogue assessment. It will be necessary to explain why further assessment has to be carried out and why procedures may be combined. Methods of observation and recording will need to be explained, discussed and agreed.
5. Set criteria for success in advance and define aims clearly. Many interventions are rapidly effective, and it may be necessary to stress the importance of ensuring generalization and maintaining the new behaviour. Negotiate arrangements for obtaining follow-up information, both direct and indirect.

6. Set a review date within a short period after the programme has started to allow early discussion of any difficulties that arise. If there are clear indications that the intervention is not going well, some of the steps in paragraphs 3–5 above may need to be repeated and modifications made.

It may be important to reassure parents and teachers that the long-term adjustment of children who have been selectively mute appears in most cases to be satisfactory, even if they remain quiet and socially inhibited personalities. It is important to clarify the arrangements and access for further advice and help.

There has been no large-scale study of the effectiveness of different approaches to the treatment of selective mutism. The rarity of the condition places difficulties in the way of such a study (see next chapter), but our review of the substantial literature of individual case reports has led us to conclude that the staged procedure described above has a number of advantages. It will facilitate approaches to treatments that:

- minimize disruption for the family and the school.
- are cost-effective in terms of time.
- are relatively likely to meet with success.

The procedure is not a panacea. Working through the sequence mechanically will not bring success. As in all behavioural work, success depends partly on skills of empathy and communication that do not appear in the treatment model but are crucial to the social process through which it is implemented.

Chapter 8
Contemporary combined approaches

In Chapters 1–3 we provided evidence that selective mutism is a multi-faceted phenomenon which probably has roots in individual differences of temperament but develops and is maintained through interactions between the individual, the family and the community. In Chapters 4–7 we showed that single educational and therapeutic interventions may often be effective in enabling children to overcome their inhibitions against speaking in certain settings. However, some children do not respond to changes in educational regime or behavioural programmes or any other single approach. In this chapter we will examine the contribution that can be made by combined approaches, including approaches that employ psychopharmacology as one element in the therapeutic strategy. If a child's pattern of selective mutism is multiply determined or has been established over a long period of their growth and development, there are good reasons to believe that combined approaches will be more likely to be effective in addressing all the barriers to relaxed communication across settings.

Although it is only recently that workers in this field have developed a clear rationale for combining particular intervention approaches, it was not uncommon for earlier writers to report the employment of a range of approaches in different combinations. Thus, for example, Ciottone and Madonna (1984) described an 'ecological' intervention that incorporated individual counselling, video role play, group work and stimulus fading. They justified the ecological label because they had tried 'to treat not only the mute child as an individual entity but to involve many aspects of his environment (i.e. locations and people)' (p. 24). As noted in the discussion of family therapy in Chapter 5, family work has often been combined with a behavioural intervention focused on the child (e.g. by Rosenberg and Lindblad, 1978).

A sustained initiative to develop a combined approach to the treatment of selective mutism has been reported in a series of four papers over a period of almost 30 years by Wright (1968), Wright et al. (1985), Krohn, Weckstein and Wright (1992) and Weckstein, Krohn and Wright (1995)

associated with the Hawthorn Center in Northville, Missouri. Their technique was based on a view of the condition which highlights 'an
underlying angry oppositional stance frequently occurring in response to
an overenmeshed maternal-child relationship' (Krohn, Weckstein and
Wright, 1992, p. 717). At the same time it was appreciated that 'despite the
child's resistance, the child is very ambivalent about his symptoms'
(Weckstein, Krohn and Wright, 1995, p. 193). As described in the 1992
paper, the approach combined a number of elements, each of which the
team saw as essential:

- The initial contact involves a thorough psychiatric evaluation, including
  developmental, familial and medical factors.
- Parents are taught about the syndrome with an emphasis on the damaging effects on development if a child is allowed to continue
  withholding speech.
- The clinician has an individual interview with the child in which they
  try to establish a strong rapport, partly by demonstrating empathy with
  the condition.
- After scheduling a complete day in agreement with the parents, the clinician meets the child alone and demands that he or she speaks before
  leaving the meeting. 'Most children speak within 1 to 2 hours, and
  rarely are more than 4 hours necessary.' (p. 713) The therapist and subsequently the parents praise the child generously when they cross that
  threshold, which may involve speaking just a single word aloud.
- Parents are then advised to require the child to speak for themselves in
  public, e.g. when ordering a meal in a restaurant with the family. If they
  have difficulty in following through this task, this may indicate that family work is needed.
- Soon after the child has begun speaking in the clinic similar firm steps
  are taken to require speech in the school setting.

Thus the intervention will involve active work in a carefully scheduled
sequence across settings and people with whom the child interacts. The
approach is based on a clear view of the aetiology of selective mutism and
aims to unpick each of the strands that ties the child to a particular pattern of communication. The aetiological model is currently
unfashionable; recent evidence does not support it, and Wright himself
has begun to adopt a more cautious view of how oppositional behaviour
should be interpreted (Wright, 1994). Most importantly, there are harsh
elements in the strategy that many therapists will find unacceptable.
Nonetheless it must be recorded that the clinical team reported a high
rate of success, describing the treatment outcome as 'at least fair in all
cases and excellent for 85%' (p. 711). However, these figures are based on
a subset of 20 cases. There were originally 29 in the series that they
reviewed. Four families were referred elsewhere for treatment, (e.g.
because of the distance of their home from the centre), but five refused

or discontinued treatment. This approach may not have been as comprehensively successful as the authors appear to have claimed, and it does not accord with current thinking on the aetiology of selective mutism, but it has been described in some detail here because it combines apparently disparate elements in a carefully thought through and coherent strategy. We wish to emphasize that combination strategies for intervening in selective mutism need not be just eclectic mixtures of approaches to treatment but can represent a coherent response to a multifaceted phenomenon.

A range of disciplines may be involved in work with selectively mute children. In addition to the teachers, psychologists, psychiatrists and family therapists who have featured most often in earlier sections of this book, this chapter covers the work of speech and language therapists, paediatricians and general practitioners. We also consider the contributions that can be made by a range of adjuncts to therapy. The chapter closes with a case study of a child who was helped by a therapeutic strategy that combined a number of approaches.

Speech and language therapy

The option of speech and language therapy has received little attention in most of the recent literature. It featured more often in the early stages of work on selective mutism, and the work of speech and language therapists has been discussed in some detail in one at least of the current books on the subject (Johnson and Wintgens, 2001). In her exploratory enquiries Buck (1987) questioned three speech therapists and learned that they were rarely consulted or used in work with selectively mute children. Perhaps this is not surprising, in view of the manifest psychological character of the problem. It is interesting to note that in one case in which a speech and language therapist played a central treatment role, the greatest challenge to her came not in establishing and shaping speech but in helping the child to transfer it to the school situation. This required an extensive behavioural programme (Rosenbaum and Kellman, 1973). Other interventions by speech and language therapists have sometimes involved the application of behavioural principles with no explicit employment of a distinctive and separate expertise (e.g. Strait, 1958).

There is sometimes a reference to speech therapy in the opening section of case studies where earlier unsuccessful attempts at intervention are mentioned briefly before the authors go on triumphantly to describe their own more fruitful approach. For example, Todd (aged 9) had 37 sessions of speech therapy before admission to the hospital where Matson et al. (1979) helped him using overcorrection, modelling and reinforcement. Williamson et al. (1977a) report that Kenneth (aged 7) had received speech therapy for an articulation problem for two years prior to their treatment, 'but his low frequency of speech in the therapy situation had hindered any progress' (cf. Adams and Glasner, 1954; Lindblad-Goldberg, 1986).

An area where the specific expertise of speech and language therapists may be invaluable is in the assessment of key aspects of the overall picture – the child's speech and language functioning. Employing a largely test-based and clinic-oriented paradigm Johnson and Wintgens (2001) suggested a number of strategies that might facilitate effective assessment:

- Use indirect ways of screening to assess the need for formal testing.
- Train parents to carry out simple screening-type assessments at home.
- Ask parents to carry out simple assessments at the clinic.

An example they gave of the first strategy was that, if parents are concerned that a child's overall speech development is delayed, they can be asked to make an audio or videotape at home to enable a speech and language therapist to screen for impairment of speech or syntax. 'Videotapes are also useful for screening social skills and general communicative competence.' (p. 80) For example, Powell and Dalley (1995) reported an intervention in which at an early stage a speech pathologist evaluated a 20-minute recording of a child talking to her mother at home. This enabled the team to exclude the possibility that she had speech and language difficulties independently of her selective mutism.

Some workers have employed operant conditioning techniques in simple speech and language training programmes, of a kind similar to those used for therapy with children with autism or severe learning difficulties (cf. Lovaas et al., 1966). This has sometimes involved training the child to produce single words and formal sentences as though incapable of producing speech at all (e.g. Paniagua and Saeed, 1987; Pecukonis and Pecukonis, 1991). In reading such reports it is important to keep in mind that normal speech is in the repertoire of selectively mute children. If a training strategy is to draw more fully on their established strengths and is to address their specific difficulties more directly, it is likely to focus on the generalization of natural speech from those settings where it is currently found to the target settings where it is needed (see Chapters 6 and 7).

With all these provisos, it might still be expected that the expertise of speech and language therapists in working with communication problems would have relevance to a wider range of work with selectively mute children. For example, a significant proportion of selectively mute children present articulation problems or other specific speech difficulties (see Chapter 1). In some of these cases there is anxiety about ridicule and teasing, so that speech therapy which focused on this issue might contribute to an overall treatment plan. One of the children described by Smayling (1959) (Case F, aged 10) had had two years of unsuccessful psychiatric treatment before referral to the speech clinic. During extended speech therapy, efforts were made to avoid any semblance of a subjective approach or a psychotherapeutic situation. This child was highly intelligent. He proved to have a severe articulation defect, and the treatment included simplified explanations of the physiology of speech processes as well as conventional exercises (tailored to begin with work on whispering and slowly to move on to speech being voiced aloud at a later stage). Eventually his parents forced the issue of his talking in school as 'he can talk all right now'. In a preview of the stimulus-fading paradigm his speech therapist then accompanied him to school where he demonstrated what he had accomplished during his absences (cf. Rosenbaum and Kellman, 1973). When speech and language therapists have helped children to establish speech habits outside the classroom but not built a generalization strategy into their intervention, the effect has sometimes been that they have had success in the clinical situation but without transfer to the crucial everyday settings. (See, for example, Porjes, 1992, pp. 370–371 on work undertaken with S-1.)

In an alternative paradigm for drawing on this expertise it would be possible for children to be offered help to improve the quality of their speech after spontaneous speech has been established across settings. It is important to take account of the degree of intense self-consciousness and sensitivity that many selectively mute children show. Whispering may be a sign of this. In some cases attention to the quality of the child's speech may have a valuable contribution to make as one element of an overall treatment plan. But Johnson and Wintgens (2001) argue that individual intervention to remediate impaired speech can only contribute effectively to the elimination of mutism if the mutism is 'recognized, assessed and taken into account – requiring a different approach to traditional therapy' (p. 12).

In multimodal work in a residential setting with three children who had severe learning difficulties Russell, Raj and John (1998) employed speech and language therapy for specific purposes – to improve one child's articulation and to shape the mouth movements of all the children. In another account of a multidisciplinary intervention Giddan et al. (1997) described how the team's speech and language pathologist guided the core programme for an 8-year-old girl with a long-standing problem of selective mutism. Once some non-verbal communication had been established, she was taken through a staged progression through written messages, gestures and private tape recordings towards whispering, soft-voice and eventually full-voice speaking in school and beyond school.

How will speech and language therapy with selectively mute children differ from other work by this group of therapists? Johnson and Wintgens (2001) adapted the process but not the setting. First, they suggested, the child would participate less in expressive tasks during clinic sessions. Secondly, homework would play a greater part in the process, with much of the work being done by the parent or carer who accompanies the child to the clinic. 'The sessions need to be viewed as training sessions, passing on to the parent or carer the skills of the therapist. Work needs to be broken down into very small steps. The parent needs to have fully understood what they are aiming at, and to be keen to try it with their child at home' (p. 197). An alternative intervention strategy is to base the speech and language therapy programme in the home or in a setting where speech is normally found. A parent or carer with whom the child talks easily in that setting may still be the main direct agent for the work. But the ultimate stimulus-fading and generalization process will be less challenging.

In principle, the work of speech and language therapists with a multi-disciplinary team could extend beyond a focus on quality of speech, but this has rarely been demonstrated in the recent literature on selective mutism. One exception was Roe (1993) who combined ideas and techniques drawn from speech and language therapy with elements from music, movement and drama therapy in an experimental interactive therapy group to help a small group of children in an inner-city infant school who were withdrawn or selectively mute. Similarly, Tittnich (1990) reported the involvement of a speech and language pathologist in assisting teachers in a daycare programme to develop an intervention package for a 3-year-old girl who did not speak there unless her mother was present. A survey of speech and language therapists in Ireland indicated that they were more likely to adopt a communication skills approach than other approaches (Carmody, 1999).

As noted above, a crucial step in such interventions is generalization of speaking behaviour from the special setting in which it is facilitated to everyday settings where the child has not normally been speaking. Johnson and Wintgens (2001) recognized the importance of this challenge and suggested how to create the best environment for such generalization – an environment in which the child's anxiety level is reduced as far as possible. We suggest that it may be helpful if only a few people are present, if the child can see that others cannot overhear what is being said, if it is not necessary to maintain fixed eye contact with others, and if the conversation takes place in the context of an activity or game in which the visual focus is equipment or materials rather than the person/people the child is talking to. For example, Michael, who was described in Chapter 7, found it easy to speak to his mother and a psychologist in the school after hours while writing and drawing on a classroom blackboard with his sister.

An example of the involvement of a speech and language therapist as lead worker in a case was reported by Watson (1995). The intervention, which was undertaken in a special school over an extended period, was based on 'hierarchical' stages of therapy, gradually involving others in activities and gradually changing locations. Watson's sensitive collaboration with teachers was described in Chapter 4. She described her intervention as 'client led, planned largely by feel' and was concerned that she might raise expectations in staff and parents which were not then met.

AJ, aged 10, attended a school for children with moderate learning difficulties and had been mute there for a number of years. Her parents had gradually become aware of her mutism when the family were living abroad where AJ had attended a nursery and international school from 3 to 6 years of age. She had been born prematurely with perinatal complications. Developmental milestones, including language, had been delayed. Both Spanish and English were used in the home in her early years. Watson began working with her when she was 10. At school she was communicative non-verbally, nodding and shaking her head, and making eye contact. She did not use formal signing, although this had been introduced in the school. Her verbal comprehension was delayed but adequate for conversation and the demands of the curriculum. A tape recording made for her teacher showed that she had delayed but functionally adequate expressive language skills.

The first two stages of therapy were spread over seven terms and comprised:

- desensitization to **being heard on tape**, starting from easy activities and going on to reading, giving instructions and shouting
- desensitization to **communicating** (including miming and signing, drawing feelings and writing in a message book).

With hindsight, Watson felt that this might have been done more quickly, but the very gradual approach maintained the confidence of parents, staff and therapist.

From term 5 the actual use of AJ's voice in school started with putting symbolic noises on tape in school, sometimes with sound effects for ghost stories made up by the therapist. This was extended into speech sounds, beginning with nonsense words, and then using AJ as a helper with a boy doing phonological work. Single words for labelling were introduced, and then more difficult words for directing activities and the use of greetings. Desensitization included videotaping AJ's activities for others to see. AJ practised using the telephone from home with the help of AJ's parents, though this was not easy as it was prearranged, and therefore lacked real content.

From term 8 all work was taking place in AJ's classroom, both with and without support from Watson. This included reading aloud and answering questions, doing surveys round the school and discussions about the purposes of talking. By term 10 AJ was able to join a group working on the social use of language where she was one of the more able members. She was also prepared for her work experience in an infants' school by a 'dry run' in a supported visit to another infants' school. During her final year at school AJ had a second successful placement in a large department store and began to attend college; she felt it would be easier to talk there as people did not know of her previous difficulties. Watson concluded that AJ was now able to use her language skills to function independently in a variety of settings. More importantly 'she no longer perceives herself as someone who does not speak in certain settings, but as someone who is sometimes shy – a description which applies after all to many of us' (p. 174). A key factor in the progress made with this client was the effective collaboration with her teachers.

Adjuncts to therapy

Therapists in different traditions have made use of a wide variety of adjuncts to therapy which have a particular relevance to work with selectively mute children. The most common have been those aids mentioned earlier that enable people to communicate without looking directly at each other, e.g. the telephone, puppets, masks, audiotaping, and videotaping. It may be helpful here to outline some adjuncts to therapy that have been used less frequently in this work but may have a specific contribution to make in some cases of selective mutism.

With the development of microelectronic aids inside toys therapists have been able to use increasingly sophisticated aids in their work. For example, Sluckin (2000) described a battery-operated toy in the shape of an apple, which was used in an intervention with Davida (aged 8) who was initially seen at home. Davida took to this toy which ejected a worm when spoken to.

> After several sessions at home it was agreed that they would show the apple and the worm to the other children in her class. During a school visit jointly with the mother, all the children in chorus made the worm emerge from the apple. Then Davida and her mother jointly 'spoke' to the worm, and finally Davida worked the mechanism alone. The children were pleasantly surprised to hear Davida's voice for the first time, and praised her. From then on, encouraged by a sympathetic teacher, Davida started to speak in class. (p. 278)

Kee et al. (2001) reported the use of a different electronic communication device which recorded single words that the child could then play aloud in situations where he was not able to speak personally.

One aid that is not often used is the family pet. Southworth (1987, 1988) found as a classroom teacher that the first sound that a selectively mute boy in her class spoke aloud in her presence was an imitation of the 'woof' his puppy made at home. In Chapter 4 we described the role of a cockatiel in the progress made by 3-year-old Sonia. In Chapter 5 we gave an account of how Sara, an adolescent with a more entrenched pattern of selective mutism, was helped by a strategy of making tape recordings of her pet parakeet (Roberts, 1984). There has been little work of this kind, but it has been suggested that pet-facilitated therapy could play a role in work with a larger proportion of selectively mute children. Hadley (1994, Chapter 22) outlines key features of this approach to treatment.

Since the children are often so tense when challenged to speak in target settings, it might be expected that relaxation methods could be of help to them. Bozigar and Hansen (1984) made relaxation techniques and

deep breathing exercises a regular part of the ritual of their group sessions with four selectively mute children. The first report of a use of
hypnosis was negative (Tramer, 1934 cited by Haskell, 1964), and there
have been no detailed accounts of the successful use of hypnosis subsequently. But Goll (1979) offers a short positive report of an informal
intervention by an amateur hypnotist that helped one child a great deal.
In the first edition of this book nearly 10 years ago we anticipated that
'with the growing interest in the use of hypnosis with children by psychologists it is possible that the potential contribution of this technique
for work with selective mutism will be explored more fully in future
years'. During the preparation of this edition we have carried out a review
of the recent literature and have consulted colleagues with an interest in
this mode of therapy through an Internet news group. We have not been
able to trace any new published accounts of the use of hypnosis as an
adjunct to therapy in the treatment of selective mutism.

Psychopharmacology

Until the beginning of the last decade the use of medication rarely featured in efforts to help children with selective mutism. There was a broad
consensus that this was a psychological phenomenon best treated by psychological means. However, even in the early period there was one
isolated report of a punitive attempt to employ drugs as an adjunct to
treatment. Shaw (1971) initially employed intravenous injections to help
Wilma (aged 10) as an inpatient to 'overcome her presumably strong inhibitions regarding speech'. Progress was slow, but the workers noticed that
the main effect of the injections was that Wilma regarded them as a kind
of punishment for not speaking – a punishment that she would try to
avoid by producing minimal speech. Shaw continued the injection programme on the basis that Wilma could avoid a morning dosage if she met
certain speech requirements by bedtime the previous day. The requirements were slowly and systematically increased. In effect the medication
was used as a threat rather than for its intrinsic medical effects.

When researchers and clinicians began to explore the potential contribution of psychopharmacology more systematically, it was initially
suggested that the greatest value of medication in this context might come
not just from efforts to control anxiety and induce relaxation but also
from an indirect impact on talkativeness. In the first report with this focus
Golwyn and Weinstock (1990) describe the use of phenelzine with Mary
(aged 7). They had noted that other patients became garrulous when taking phenelzine (which is said to have a dopaminergic effect promoting
social engagement). Mary put on a good deal of weight and suffered from
mild (controllable) constipation as side effects. After 18 weeks the dosage
was tapered and eventually withdrawn altogether after 24 weeks. At
follow-up after 5 months the mutism had not recurred. The authors

speculated that dopaminergic systems may regulate talkativeness as well as movement and activity in diverse conditions such as parkinsonism and social phobia.

Since that report there has been an upsurge of interest in the use of medication in the treatment of selective mutism (see reviews by Campbell and Cueva, 1995; Dow et al., 1995; Pine and Grun, 1998). This has been reflected in the professional press on both sides of the Atlantic through letters and informal case studies written by individual practitioners (e.g. Boon, 1994; Jelley, 2000). In a postal survey of child and adolescent psychiatrists in the USA during 1993, Carlson, Kratochwill and Johnston (1994) found that a third of those who had treated a child with selective mutism had used psychotropic medication for the purpose. Antidepressants were the most frequently endorsed medication, with antianxiety agents mentioned by a smaller proportion of the sample. The authors concluded that, even though there were then no published reports of adequate efficacy studies, a variety of medications was being prescribed for selective mutism. They called for further research and dissemination of information in this area.

From the summary of reports on psychopharmacological studies in Table 8.1 it will be seen that there has subsequently been a steep increase in more carefully controlled research. The focus of most of these reports has been on the reduction of anxiety levels rather than on influencing systems that regulate talkativeness, as Golwyn and Weinstock suggested at the beginning of the decade. Phenelzine has been found to have undesirable side effects with children (e.g. Leonard and Topol, 1993, p. 702) and is therefore not recommended as the medication of first choice (Golwyn and Sevlie, 1999). Reviewers have concluded that the small number of controlled studies tend to favour selective serotonin reuptake inhibitors (SSRIs) both in terms of their efficacy in reducing target symptoms and their comparative lack of side effects (Pine and Grun, 1998). Some have also argued that SSRIs should be considered only when a child with selective mutism presents also with symptoms of social phobia or anxiety disorder (Dow et al., 1995; Pine and Grun, 1998). There is a striking discordance within the literature between those who appear to be ready to turn to medication as a treatment of choice in most circumstances and those who, although accepting that medication may be necessary in cases where psychosocial interventions have failed, advise against 'the indiscriminate use of psychotropic agents as a first line of treatment' (Phelps, Brown and Power, 2002). Few would go as far as Anstendig (1999) who concluded that 'small-scale studies demonstrating the effectiveness of the medication have paved the way for using fluoxetine as an essential component to intervention with selectively mute children' (p. 425). There is a need for further double-blind group studies with children across a broader age range presenting with a wider range of other symptoms before most commentators will be satisfied with so strong a conclusion.

Table 8.1 Reports of trials of drug therapy for selective mutism

Authors	Medication	Design of study	Participants	Side effects	Outcome	Follow-up
Golwyn and Weinstock (1990)	Phenelzine (built up to 60 mg/day and withdrawn after 24 weeks)	Individual case study. No other treatment	7-year-old girl	Mild constipation and weight gain	Successful treatment completed in 24 weeks	Mutism had not recurred at follow-up after 5 months
Black and Uhde (1992)	Placebo for 3 weeks, desipramine for 10 weeks, then fluoxetine (dosage built up to 20mg/day)	Individual case study with placebo control. No other treatment	12-year-old girl	No reference to side effects in the report	No effect from placebo or desipramine. With fluoxetine spoke freely to adults and peers at school after 4 weeks	All gains maintained at follow-up after 7 months
Black and Uhde (1994)	Placebo for 2 weeks, then fluoxetine or placebo for 12 weeks (dosage built up to 0.24mL/kg/day)	Double-blind group study with placebo control. No other treatment	15 children (mean age 8–9 yrs) of whom 6 were randomly selected for fluoxetine group	'The side effects were more benign than those reported in some previous studies of fluoxetine treatment ... perhaps due to (using) relatively lower doses' (p. 1006)	Fluoxetine group rated significantly more improved than placebo group by parents, but difference not significant for ratings by teachers and clinicians	No report
Motavalli (1995)	Placebo for 13 days, then fluoxetine for 6 weeks (dosage began with 20mg/day)	Individual case study with placebo control. No other treatment	12-year-old girl	'No side effects were reported.'	No effect from placebo. With fluoxetine began to speak to family members after 2 weeks	Talking and social interaction maintained and extended at regular follow-up over 12 month period.

Table 8.1 Reports of trials of drug therapy for selective mutism

Authors	Medication	Design of study	Participants	Side effects	Outcome	Follow-up
Wright et al. (1995)	Fluoxetine (4 mg/day, then 12 mg/day) added to treatment regime after 6 months with limited progress. Medication continued for over a year	Individual case study. Special day programme, individual therapy, and parents' group work as well as medication	Girl aged 4 yrs 10 months	'She has not experienced any adverse medication effects.' But researchers noted that oppositional behaviour increased	Began talking more freely in familiar situations after 5 days. By day 20 was talking freely in all settings	Continuing on the medication and with monthly family therapy one year later, is talking freely in all settings with good 'academic and behavioural progress'
Dummit et al. (1996)	Fluoxetine for 9 weeks (building up from 1.2 mg/day to 20 mg/day, then, if not improved, to 60mg/day	Open group study. Throughout the drug trial supportive counselling provided	21 children aged 5–14 yrs (16 girls and 5 boys)	2 children discontinued because of behavioural disinhibition. 9 children (43%) reported physical side effects	16 children 'improved' overall on structured assessment scales. Treatment success lower among older children	No follow-up. But authors concluded that showing the full clinical effects may require trial longer than 9 weeks
Guna-Dumitrescu and Pelletier (1996)	Fluoxetine (20 mg/day, then 30 mg/day). Duration not reported	Individual case study. Hospital inpatient, behaviour programme including shaping and escape procedures as well as medication	8-year-old boy	No reference to side effects in the report	No improvement after 4 weeks of medication on its own. With multimodal treatment began to speak after 3 weeks	Communication generalized rapidly and was speaking in all social situations on follow-up

Table 8.1 Reports of trials of drug therapy for selective mutism

Authors	Medication	Design of study	Participants	Side effects	Outcome	Follow-up
Kehle et al. (1998)	Fluoxetine (10 mg/day for 4 weeks, then 20 mg/day for unspecified period)	Individual case study. Medication used to augment video self-modelling	9-year-old girl (one of three case studies in this report)	No reference to side effects in the report	Restricted speech after 3 weeks of video self-modelling intervention. Speech 'dramatically improved' with fluoxetine (20mg/day)	'Treatment effects were maintained' at 9 month follow-up.
Russell, Raj and John (1998)	2/3 children who did not improve with other treatments given fluoxetine (5 mg/day for 7 days, then 10 mg/day)	Individual case study. Multimodal residential therapy programme including behaviour plan, speech therapy and stimulus fading	3 children with mental retardation. Ages not given	No reference to side effects in the report	'Clinical and statistical improvement sustained throughout the 12 weeks of study.'	No follow-up reported
Lafferty and Constantino (1998)	Fluvoxamine (50 mg/day, 100 mg/day, and then alternating dosages). Discontinued after 6 months	Individual case study. No other treatment Previously had had psychotherapy without success	6-year-old girl with obsessive-compulsive traits as well as SM	Hyperactivity, untidiness (out of character for her), decreased sleep, distractibility	Began speaking in school 2 days after dosage increased to 100 mg/day	SM resolved but oppositional behaviour at home continued after 9 months

Table 8.1 Reports of trials of drug therapy for selective mutism

Authors	Medication	Design of study	Participants	Side effects	Outcome	Follow-up
Carlson, Kratochwill and Johnston (1994)	No medication for 2 weeks, placebo for at least 2 weeks and 50mg or 100mg/ day sertraline for 8–12 weeks	Double-blind group study with placebo control No other treatment	5 children aged 5–11 yrs	'Minimal side effects were reported.' One child had passing problems with insomnia	2/5 participants free of symptoms after <10 weeks sertraline treatment, but group results variable	Follow-up at 20 weeks showed a third participant to be without symptoms
Hagerman et al. (1999)	Fluoxetine (10 mg/day later increased to 20 mg/day)	Individual case study. Simultaneous psychological therapy	12-year-old girl	No side effects with 10 mg dosage. No report on impact of 20 mg	Increased talking with some but not all target people. Improved mood, reduced anxiety	Work was continuing at the time when the report was published
Rupp (1999)	Fluoxetine (5 mg/day increased gradually to 20 mg/day). Clonidine added and withdrawn. Then haloperidol (0.5 mg twice daily)	Individual case study. No other treatment Previously had had play therapy and a behavioural plan without success	5-year-old girl who displayed aggression and motor and vocal tics with SM	Clonidine 'caused sedation and interfered with school functioning'. No side effects reported in association with fluoxetine	Improved non-verbal communication after 2 months' fluoxetine, spontaneous speech with extended family after 3 months	After 8 months regressed in aggressive behaviour and tics. With haloperidol these improved. After 1 month speaking at home, school and clinic
Golwyn and Sevlie (1999)	Phenelzine in varying doses for each child. Replacing fluoxetine for one child	Individual case studies. Varying treatment methods had previously been attempted	4 children aged 4–7 yrs	Side effects varied and included mild constipation, weight gain, sleep disturbance	Improved spontaneous speaking in all cases and amelioration of some other symptoms	Dosages tapered over periods of some months and improvements monitored

Table 8.1 Reports of trials of drug therapy for selective mutism

Authors	Medication	Design of study	Participants	Side effects	Outcome	Follow-up
Kee et al. (2001)	Fluoxetine (10mg/day, later increased to 30 mg/day)	Individual case study. With systematic desensitization using an electronic communication device	9-year-old boy	None reported	Spoke to a stranger in public and read aloud in his remedial teacher's hearing	Treatment continuing at the time of the report
Maskey (2001)	Moclobemide (75 mg twice daily for 2 weeks, then 150 mg)	Individual case study. Hospital inpatient treatment with behaviour management and family therapy	12-year-old girl who had been selectively mute since age of 6	'There were no adverse effects reported . . . (she) liked taking the medication as it made her feel less anxious.'	Significant (though uneven) increases in word frequency and utterance frequency	Progress not maintained after discharge

A disappointing feature of the reports summarized in Table 8.1 is that psychopharmacological treatment is not often combined with other interventions. The reports by Wright et al. (1995), Guna-Dumitrescu and Pelletier (1996), Dummit et al. (1996), Kehle et al. (1998), Hagerman et al. (1999), Russell, Raj and John (1998), Kee et al. (2001) and Maskey (2001) are exceptions to this. As we argued above, there are good reasons for developing combined and multimodal forms of intervention for selective mutism.

Combined approaches

An increasing proportion of the case study reports being published describe combined approaches to intervention with multidisciplinary teamwork. Investigators who had reported single modes of intervention previously have been more likely in the last 15 years to employ a multimodal approach (e.g. Kehle et al., 1998), and those who had been employing multimodal approaches for some time extended the range of combinations in their repertoire (e.g. Wright et al., 1995). Clinic-based therapists have explored new ways of supporting changes in the behavioural environment in schools, as illustrated in Chapter 4. Those engaged in school-based work have drawn upon clinical collaborators much more extensively. For example, Giddan et al. (1997) describe an intervention strategy with an 8-year-old girl, Mimi, who had resisted earlier attempts at treatment which involved individual psychotherapy once a week and speech-language therapy twice a week (with peers joining in when Mimi was ready) plus behaviour modification in the classroom based on a token economy system. Work with her parents included quarterly team review conferences in which changing treatment goals were established. This team favoured the use of multiple sites for intervention with varied interventions across sites, but they worked hard to ensure that the professionals' efforts were coordinated, that they maintained consistent reward systems and complemented each others' programmes.

Dow et al. (1995) advocated a 'school-based multidisciplinary individualized treatment plan' and at the same time argued that different clinical approaches could be 'integrated to decrease anxiety and to encourage speech and social interaction' (pp. 844–846). An example of work along these lines is given in Chapter 4 where we described intervention for Will who was just starting at secondary school. He was successfully helped through a combination of behavioural approaches, medication and ongoing support for staff at the school. This example reinforced the point made at the beginning of this chapter – that, although a single educational and therapeutic intervention may be successful with some selectively mute children, there are situations where a combined approach may be the most effective strategy. It seems likely that this will be particularly valuable when a child's pattern of selective mutism is multiply determined or has been established over a long period.

Chapter 9
Research

In the book so far we have quoted research reports frequently but have not analysed the challenges and opportunities that are presented to researchers working in this field. There are particular problems caused by the low incidence of selective mutism. In this chapter we consider some of the methodological issues raised by published surveys and studies of substantial samples of children and also examine the methodology of individual case studies, single-case research designs and follow-up studies. Ultimately, improvements in the assessment and treatment of selective mutism depend on high-quality research into successful clinical and educational practice.

Studies of substantial samples of children

Because selective mutism is rare, there have been very few studies in which investigators have had access to substantial samples of children. No published studies bring together data on children across a large geographical area. As noted in Chapter 1, most reports that cover more than one or two children review a series who had been seen in a particular centre or by a particular worker over a period of years. A summary of the sample sizes in published reports in English up to 1993 is given in Table 9.1. It appears that 90% of the reports published during that period concerned fewer than 10 children and 64% concerned a single case.

Table 9.1 Sample size in studies of selective mutism published in English up to 1993

Sample size	1	2–3	4–6	7–9	10+
No. of reports	62	16	8	1	10

Over the past 10 years there have been more group studies. An updated analysis of the largest reported clinical samples is given in Table 9.2.

Table 9.2 Clinical and other studies with a sample size of 10+ in chronological order

	Sample	Source	Definition
Parker, Olsen and Throckmorton (1960)	27	School social work programme in one area	No
Wright (1968)	24	One clinic	No
Friedman and Karagan (1973)	13	Clinics of one university	No
Koch and Goodlund (1973)	13	One inpatient facility	No
Goll (1979)	10	Two workers in separate clinics	No
Lowenstein (1979)	21	Referred to one educational psychologist	No
Wergeland (1979)	11	Admitted to one hospital department	No
Kolvin and Fundudis (1981)	24	All clinics in one area	Yes
Wilkins (1985)	24	One hospital department	Yes
Sluckin, Foreman and Herbert (1991)	25	Referred by schools in one area	Yes
Krohn, Weckstein and Wright (1992)	20	Treated at one clinic or in the private practice of one of the authors	Yes
Black and Uhde (1995)	30	Population survey in one area drawing on information from school counsellors	Yes
Steinhausen and Juzi (1996)	100	Referred through a parents' self-help group, a psychiatric service or a hospital department	Yes[a]
Dummit et al. (1997)[b]	50	Recruited through local schools and the Selective Mutism Foundation Inc.	Yes
Ford et al. (1998)	153	Postal survey to those on the mailing list of the Selective Mutism Foundation Inc.	Yes[c]
Andersson and Thomsen (1998)	37	One hospital department	Yes[a]
Kumpulainen et al. (1998)	38	Population study of second grade pupils in a Finnish county	Yes
Kristensen (2002)	54	Survey based on referrals from child psychiatry clinics and school psychology services throughout Norway	Yes

[a] These authors employed ICD-10 criteria (WHO, 1992) for selective mutism.
[b] Dummit et al. (1996) report on the treatment of a subgroup of the children reported on in their 1997 article, so the 1996 reference is not listed separately here.
[c] These authors queried the DSM-IV definition on the basis of their study.

The question answered in the final column of this table was – is there evidence that a clear definition of selective mutism was adopted consistently when deciding whether or not to include children in the sample? It will be seen that in the earlier reports there are frequently problems in ascertaining whether investigators employed consistent criteria in defining cases of selective mutism. Even when a consistent definition was employed, there may be difficulties. The report on 68 children by Hayden (1980) was excluded from the table, because the definition that she used was idiosyncratic to herself and was wider and looser than the normally accepted definition. For example, the mute behaviour had to persist for only 8 weeks for a child to be included in the sample.

In most of the early published reports the reviews covered cases seen over a wide time span, and little detail was provided about arrangements to ensure consistency in information sources. Wilkins (1985) studied case files from one hospital department over a period of 12 years, Wright (1968) looked back at cases he himself had worked with over 7 years, and Goll (1979) mixed these two methods, spanning a shorter but undefined period. Only Kolvin and Fundudis (1981) sought specified information in a consistent format from a range of workers in an area, focusing on the relatively recent past. During that period the literature had no concurrent study of cases being seen at the time of the investigation by professionals across a wide area. When we wrote the first edition of this book 10 years ago, we argued that that approach would be the only viable one with a phenomenon as rare as selective mutism, if investigators were to achieve greater consistency of definition and information on a substantial study sample.

Surveys of the kind carried out by Brown and Lloyd (1975), Bradley and Sloman (1975) and Cline and Kysel (1987/88) made a contribution to identifying key characteristics of the selectively mute population. The first of these studies helped to chart the course of recovery from initial shyness after starting school. All three studies highlighted the issue of ethnic minority overrepresentation. But surveys of this kind face problems of definition too. For example, it is not possible to be sure that the headteachers whose returns were analysed by Cline and Kysel (1987/88) employed the term 'elective mutism' in a consistent way. More important, improvements in strategies for helping selectively mute children cannot be studied through such methods. Because of the rarity of the phenomenon, it is doubtful that it would be possible to generalize from a small group on the assumption that it was representative of the whole population of selectively mute children. It is not surprising, then, that most of the early advances in understanding and treating the children depended on the detailed analysis of individual cases.

In recent years, as Table 9.2 shows, there has been a sharp increase in the number of studies with substantial group sizes. There have been undoubted gains from this trend, but the findings of such studies have to be evaluated in the light of their methodological limitations too. Firstly, the collection of data is based on individual judgements of a large number of people who may well be inconsistent in how they interpret what is required of them. Secondly, enquiries tend to be more superficial because there are no means of exploring issues in depth case by case. Thirdly, there are often problems of sampling bias. For example, Ford et al. (1998) undertook a careful postal survey of 153 respondents from the mailing list of the Selective Mutism Foundation. With justification they claimed that this was the 'largest sample of SM ever studied' and the first to have 'included people from all four regions of the United States' (p. 195). At the same time they had to acknowledge that the response rate to the survey was only 48% and that people contacting the Selective Mutism Foundation are almost certainly not a representative sample of all those whose children are selectively mute. For example, nearly three quarters of the respondents reported that selective mutism had persisted for 3 years or more – a higher proportion than in other studies. They concluded that 'we must be cautious about generalizing the results to clinic-based SM populations' (p. 222). However, in spite of all the reasons for caution, studies of larger samples of selectively mute children have made an increasingly important contribution to our understanding of the phenomenon in recent years. For that reason we have cited reports on these studies many times in this book. In the future it is to be hoped that the value of such studies can be further enhanced by ensuring that the samples that are studied are more representative of selective mutism across society and by including comparisons between people who are selectively mute and controls who are not.

Individual case studies

The individual case study is often treated dismissively in textbooks of scientific method in psychology. It may be seen as a useful source of ideas and hypotheses, but it is not seen as a valid basis for scientific generalization. The key problem for most commentators is that it is not possible to specify the conditions under which what is discovered about a single case holds true of a whole population. In addition, many of those who have reported case studies in the past have violated fundamental scientific principles in the way they collected and analysed their data and in the way they interpreted and reported on their findings. A major proponent of case study research has acknowledged: 'Too many times the case study investigator has been sloppy and has allowed equivocal evidence or biased views to influence the direction of the findings and conclusions' (Yin, 1994). Examples of poor practice of this kind abound in the literature on selective mutism. Very often rich and fascinating reports by respected practitioners have failed to specify key factors in their accounts so that it is not possible to know exactly how children presented at the outset, or what was done to help them, or how their behaviour changed over time and in different settings.

However, when case study methods are practised with greater rigour, there seems little doubt that they can make a substantial contribution to our understanding of selective mutism. This is not just a counsel of despair, on the grounds that the phenomenon is rare so that it is very difficult to assemble representative samples. There are other reasons, too, for seeing the case study approach as particularly valuable in this field. The model of selective mutism presented in Chapter 3 highlighted an interaction between the child, the family and the community, and Yin defined the case study method of enquiry in the following terms. This method 'investigates a contemporary phenomenon within its real-life context, when the boundaries between phenomenon and context are not clearly evident, and in which multiple sources of evidence are used'.

A rigorous case study approach could play an important part in evaluating a multi-level model of selective mutism and in identifying key developmental and social factors associated with ethnic and gender over-representation. In each case generalization from single case studies will be possible if inferences are drawn to a theory (the process of *analytical generalization*) and not to a population (the process of *statistical generalization*). The enquiry must be designed to enable the investigator to test specific predictions from a particular theory (Yin, 1994; Bassey, 1999). As in the design of any scientific experiment, a case may be analysed to test differential predictions from rival theories. An example of success within this paradigm is the report on a single case by Croghan and Craven (1982). They presented what could be seen as a critical case for testing Reed's (1963) hypothesis that selectively mute children fall into two distinct groups. They showed that JB (aged 8) was not only manipulative but also highly anxious: only when her anxiety was fully appreciated and treated was it possible for her to speak in a relaxed way in school.

It is important to be clear what kinds of conclusion may be drawn from a case study of that kind. JB represented a counterinstance of a generalization that had been seen as universally applicable. The evidence of a single case can thus 'cast doubt on a general proposition'. But it cannot in itself 'allow affirmative claims of a very general nature to be made' (Kazdin, 1992). It would require repeated demonstrations of the same phenomenon for an affirmative generalization to be put forward with confidence. That is what has happened in this instance, as a number of other case studies have shown that evidence of underlying anxiety often accompanies manipulative behaviour in selectively mute children (see Chapter 2). A single case study cannot on its own offer sufficient evidence to support an affirmative generalization, but a series of single case studies, all pointing in the same direction, may offer strong support. They will not together constitute a 'sample' of the population, but each will constitute a replication of the original finding. Successive studies may replicate the first by predicting the same result in similar circumstances (*literal replication*). Alternatively, they may demonstrate different results in conditions in which the theory that is being tested predicts the difference (*theoretical replication*).

How can one be sure that a single case study report is valid? Table 9.3 lists a number of strategies proposed by Yin (1994) for collecting and analysing evidence in case study research in order to maintain high scientific principles. Space does not allow a full discussion here of the methods listed in this table, and readers are referred to Yin's text.

Table 9.3 Strategies for the conduct of case study research

Data collection	Data analysis
Use multiple sources of evidence	Match the pattern of data that are found with a predicted pattern (or with several alternative predictions)
Create a case study database	Build an explanation for the data by stipulating a set of causal links about it and consider the possibility of rival explanations
Maintain a chain of evidence	Record specific indicators at specific time intervals over a period and conduct a time series analysis

From Yin (1994).

One strategy for getting round the problems of single case study research is to combine the results of many such studies through systematic meta-analysis (Busk and Serlin, 1992). This replaces the methods employed in traditional *narrative* reviews. Instead, investigators undertake a *quantitative* synthesis of the available evidence. The aim is that the analysis will systematically take account of the methodological quality of each empirical report that is available and of the size of any effect or difference that is associated with, say, differences in treatment regime. Only one such analysis has been attempted in selective mutism research – a 'best evidence synthesis' of the evidence on approaches to treatment (Stone et al., 2002). The conclusions of their report were summarized in Chapter 6. They confirmed the findings of earlier reviewers that treatment, including specifically behaviourally oriented treatment, has a higher rate of proven effectiveness than no treatment. Unfortunately, although the analysis of evidence in this study was more systematic than in any previous review, the conclusions that the authors were able to draw were somewhat limited. They had to employ rather broad categories of types of treatment, with the result that they could not differentiate effectively between different approaches within the behavioural tradition. Their two categories of 'applied behavioural analysis' and 'combined behavioural approaches' were not sufficiently finely drawn to make it possible to resolve major questions in the behavioural treatment of selective mutism such as those addressed through narrative review in Chapter 7 above. This is not a criticism of their strategy, but an acknowledgment of the impact of shortcomings of reporting in this field that were noted above. They had set 13 criteria to code empirical reports for method-ological quality and found that only about 30% of the cases they reviewed met 4 or more of those criteria. 'Although we expected to find differential effectiveness among four common models of behavior therapy, due to lack of quantifiable data in the other behavior therapy models (i.e. neobe-havioristic, social learning theory, and cognitive behavior therapy), we were unable to test our original prediction' (p. 184).

A systematic meta-analysis can only be as effective as the quality of the data that are synthesised. Probably the most important section of the report by Stone, Kratochwill and their colleagues was the discussion in which they suggested ways in which the quality of research design and reporting could be improved. They called for:

- more 'within group' design studies of the same treatment
- greater use of systematic treatment manuals to facilitate replication by other investigators
- more reporting of measures of treatment integrity, i.e. how closely the treatment that was given followed the planned procedure set out in the manual
- greater use of systematic assessment methods for measuring children's states before, during and after treatment, e.g. standardized behaviour rating scales or systematic observations to measure anxiety
- the use of a broader range of outcome studies, e.g. recording academ-ic achievement and measures of anxiety and phobia as well as the usual commentary on patterns of verbal communication
- more consistency across studies in the selection of outcome measures to facilitate the comparison of effect sizes between studies.

Although the substantive conclusions of this paper on treatment meth-ods in selective mutism were rather limited, it offered a very powerful analysis of the weaknesses of research methodology in this field and a persuasive list of recommendations for improvement. But the evaluation of treatment strategies is becoming more complex as the multimodal approaches to treatment that were described in Chapter 8 become more common. As Hechtman (1993) showed in the context of research into the treatment of attention deficit hyperactive disorder, we are at an early stage in identifying and overcoming the technical and practical chal-lenges that confront researchers when evaluating multimodal approaches to treatment.

Single-case research designs

When the purpose of an investigation of a single case is to decide whether or not a particular intervention was the cause of a predicted change in behaviour, there are more effective research strategies available than those described in the previous section. In this situation single-case experimental designs allow the investigator to draw valid inferences about effects on performance over time. This means that an affirmative statement can be made about the results on the basis of one case alone. These designs are closer in rationale to the traditional experimental design in which a comparison is made between groups that have been treated differently. With these designs a comparison is made between how a single subject responds when different treatments are applied: the subject is his/her own 'control' (Kazdin, 1992, Chapter 7). All the major reviews of behavioural methods for treating selective mutism advocated this form of design 20 years ago (Sanok and Ascione, 1979; Kratochwill, 1981; Cunningham et al., 1983; Labbe and Williamson, 1984). Their conclusions on such issues as behavioural assessment and the definition of outcome criteria are summarized in the section on methodology in Chapter 5. Here it is necessary to examine the options for research design in more detail.

Many investigators of selective mutism have employed AB designs (where A is the situation without any intervention and B is the intervention). Some of these have used baseline assessment involving repeated observations over a period rather than simply a one-off pre-test and post-test. That represents an improvement on traditional case study narrative accounts, but such a design is still methodologically weak because it does not rule out the possibility that any change in behaviour has occurred in response to some other factor independently of the intervention, e.g. maturation. A number of design options have been developed to overcome such problems, including three that have featured particularly in the literature on selective mutism – ABAB designs, multiple baseline designs, and changing criterion designs.

ABAB designs

In the ABAB design, treatment is alternated with no treatment over more than one cycle (a crucial difference from the AB design). It is predicted that behaviour will change during the B phases but will revert during the second A phase closer to its baseline pattern. There are some examples of its use with selectively mute children (e.g. Morin, Ladouceur and Cloutier, 1982; Watson and Kramer, 1992), but this design is not usually considered suitable for work in this context. Clinicians are properly reluctant to risk a setback once the child has begun to speak. There are also problems in interpreting this design if withdrawal of a treatment does not lead to a reversal of the target behaviour. Should one conclude that the treatment was not responsible for the change in behaviour in the first place, or can one perhaps conclude that the intervention was so effective that the desired behaviour is now well established and not affected by minor changes in contingencies? Speaking is likely to be maintained by ordinary social contingencies once it starts in a new setting.

Multiple baseline design

In one form of the multiple baseline design, data for a defined verbal response are collected across settings where the child does not speak, e.g. a classroom, a small group setting in school, and a physical education lesson. Then the intervention is applied in each setting in sequence. If the child's behaviour changes in a setting only when the intervention is made, this is taken as evidence of a specific effect of the intervention (e.g. Griffith et al., 1975; Munford et al., 1976; Sanok and Striefel, 1979; Piersel and Kratochwill, 1981; Cunningham et al., 1983; Larsson and Larsson, 1983; Pecukonis and Pecukonis, 1991; Watson and Kramer, 1992; Sheridan, Kratochwill and Ramirez, 1995). There are some difficulties in employing this design in work on selective mutism, as there are examples of cases where changing the child's verbal behaviour in one setting leads to changes in another setting without further intervention (e.g. Maria who was described in the previous chapter). For this reason, perhaps, the multiple baseline design has not been employed in this field as much as it has in research on the treatment of some other childhood behaviour problems. However, Dowrick and Hood (1978) showed that a multiple baseline design can also be applied across subjects in the rare situation in which two selectively mute children are referred at the same time. Kehle et al. (1998) argued that increasing the number of assessment occasions within as well as across settings allows valid inferences to be drawn from the results with an AB design. This does not actually address the main limitations of that design. More persuasively, they demonstrated improvements with their favoured treatment strategy across three children in three different settings.

Changing criterion design

In the changing criterion design, the intervention is carried out in phases. During each phase a set criterion is applied for the behaviour that is required in order to gain reinforcement. Once the target behaviour is well established, the treatment enters a new phase and a new criterion is set. If behaviour changes in a stepwise fashion in response to each successive change in criterion level, this is taken as evidence that it is the intervention that is causing the changes. This design is used most effectively when shaping procedures are part of the intervention and the changes that are planned are expected to be gradual in effect (eg. Crissy in Williamson et al., 1977b), but the design can be used with other approaches too (e.g. Paniagua and Saeed, 1987).

These designs allow an investigator to draw fairly confident inferences about the impact of the selected intervention technique. When investigators wish to compare the impact of different techniques on the same child (or the same techniques in different combinations), they cannot employ the same approach. Instead, they must employ a strategy which allows the effects of each combination to be examined independently. For example, in work with Emma (aged 6) Wulbert et al. (1973) were able to show that positive reinforcement did not produce verbal responses unless combined with stimulus fading. Time out for not responding was also used. This was not effective with reinforcement alone, but facilitated response if used together with stimulus fading. It has been claimed that an alternating treatment design of this kind has another advantage. 'Identifying particular techniques which have failed in the context of an ultimately successful case will help to counter the bias introduced by publication policies favoring positive outcomes' (Cunningham et al., 1983).

Follow-up of children who have been selectively mute

Over the last 25–30 years many reports of work with selectively mute children have offered detailed and systematic accounts of the interventions that were carried out and of the children's immediate response. A smaller proportion of reports have also offered a fairly systematic account of the child's pattern of communication before intervention started. But there are still very few reports which systematically cover generalization of the improvements that are achieved and subsequent follow-up. This can be seen by examining Table 6.2 which lists 33 reports on behavioural approaches published between 1982 and 2002. Nearly half of these have no follow-up report at all, and several of those that do report on follow-up present only the most cursory evidence. This seems particularly unfortunate now that we have good reason to believe that individuals who have presented a pattern of selective mutism in childhood are likely to show a significant degree of shyness and social anxiety into adolescence and adulthood (Joseph, 1999). Some therapists have followed up a series of cases that they had treated in the past (Wright, 1968; Sluckin, Foreman and Herbert, 1991), though this has rarely involved the controlled comparison of outcome for children treated in different ways (Leonard and Topol, 1993). Table 9.4 presents a selection of examples of the full follow-up data given in published individual case reports. It includes the period before 1982, partly because some detailed follow-up work was carried out in the earlier period. (See the full report of indirect observations from home and school in Scott, 1977, pp. 269–270, which was too long to reproduce in full.)

Semenoff, Park and Smith (1976) presented a detailed account of intervention with Roger who had been selectively mute since entering kindergarten. The most intensive work took place while he was in first grade. In the second grade the teacher had occasional follow-up conferences with the speech therapist, school nurse and psychologist to evaluate his progress. Regular observations were made by the psychologist as part

Table 9.4 Examples of published follow-up reports

Clayton (1981)	'This behaviour [reading aloud in class and conveying messages audibly to teachers and pupils alike] was still being maintained 9 months after completion of the programme, and appeared to be self-reinforcing. Reports from other pupils and independent post-treatment playground observation by the psychologist revealed that Clarissa was engaging in, and initiating, spontaneous conversation with other pupils and staff.'
Holmbeck and Lavigne (1992)	'At 6-month follow-up (middle of 2nd grade) Mary's mother reported that she was talking freely to her classroom and physical education teachers and several of her classmates, and was talking aloud in reading group. Her mother also reported that she had performed successfully in two piano recitals at the beginning of second grade. On the other hand, she was still uncomfortable talking aloud to the entire class; her teacher reported that she would still whisper when in a large group setting.'
Kehle, Owen and Cressy (1990)	'We also brought the formerly mute child to the University to discuss his elective mutism with graduate psychology students. This 6-year-old, formerly elective mute child confidently walked into a rather large room and sat down at a table in front of approximately 25 strange adults, folded his arms and stated, 'Well, what is it you want to know?'. . . After 7 months follow-up indicated that the formerly mute child was functioning extremely well. He freely communicated verbally with his peers and faculty. He also volunteered to assist the authors with other mute children who may be in the district.'
Lazarus, Gavillo and Moore (1983)	Karen (aged 7) 'continued speaking to her classroom teacher and other students throughout the remainder of the school year. This was facilitated by adding additional students to Karen's reading group and asking classmates to direct questions to each other. The following year Karen was placed in a clinical day treatment program where she was observed speaking to her teacher, four other adults and several children. Karen is still continuing to make slow and steady progress.'
Lindblad-Goldberg (1986)	'A follow-up 2 years later indicated that Jerry had successfully completed first grade, talked with teachers and children, and participated easily in an oral reading group.'
Morin, Ladouceur and Cloutier (1982)	'The behavior modification program. . . was divided into five phases involving 22 sessions: ABABB. Each of these sessions was held on different days in the classroom. The teacher served as behavior change agent in the whole study. She asked the child an average of ten questions each session. These questions related to the daily life of the kindergarten and requested a verbal response. . . One year after the end of the treatment, the teacher and an independent observer (a graduate student in psychology) evaluated the child's verbal behavior in two additional sessions.'
Pigott and Gonzales (1987)	'In a 6-month telephone follow-up, the child's mother report ed that Chuck was making straight A's in school and had several classmates with whom he frequently talked over the phone, and she reported receiving numerous positive reports from his fourth-grade teachers.'
Richards and Hansen (1978)	'A 15-month follow-up indicated Amy was still talking regularly (>8 times/day) in class. Her fourth grade teacher even complained that she talked too much! Futhermore, Amy had volunteered to play the part of Betsy Ross in a school play. She got the part and did a fine, verbose job. A five year follow-up indicated that Amy was still regularly in school and progressing normally in terms of her school work.'

of the monitoring process (a 15-minute period of event sampling observation in the classroom twice a month). Observations from January to April that year showed that he was responding to 100% of the questions directed to him. In addition the psychologist monitored his spontaneous, initiating remarks and compared their frequency to that of the spontaneous remarks of another child in the class selected at random. Figure 9.1 shows the spontaneous speech observed during these periods.

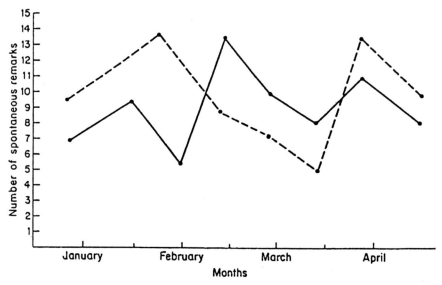

Figure 9.1 Follow-up observations in the classroom from a study of Semenoff et al. (1976), showing spontaneous speech observed during 15-minute periods. ●———● Roger, average 9; ●- - -● child at random, average 9.4

Kratochwill (1981) advocated not only that follow-up should be based on direct observation of the client, as practised by Semenoff and her colleagues, but that these observations should be made under the recording conditions established during the therapeutic programme (which was not true in Semenoff's study). He pointed out that, if the same or similar variables were used, it would be possible for the researcher to assess the progress of the child on a time continuum with the same measures of performance as during the intervention and the baseline period. Some may see the advice to employ such instruments as a counsel of perfection in the context of busy clinical duties. It is symptomatic that, when Kratochwill and his colleagues worked with a 6-year-old girl, Stacy, some years later, their positive results could not be followed up because 'the school year ended and further programming . . . could not be planned' (Sheridan, Kratochwill and Ramirez, 1995, pp. 72–73). There are many obstacles to follow-up. The school year cycle is only one. Another arises from the many pressures on the time of clinical investigators. As shown in the table, Morin and his colleagues managed a one-year follow-up only by using a graduate student in psychology as observer. At the same time it is not impossible to achieve the standards that Kratochwill set 20 years ago. For example, Watson and Kramer (1992) conducted a monthly probe of the number of words spoken by 9-year-old Tim in five different settings over a three month follow-up period. They employed the same strategy for doing so as they had done for a baseline assessment and while treatment was in progress.

As will also be seen from Table 9.4, other, less systematic strategies are possible. Kehle, Owen and Cressy (1990) drew on their own first-hand experience and selected vivid anecdotal detail which is clearly intended to convey the strength and generalizability of the child's improvement. Richards and Hansen (1978) and Clayton (1981) mixed direct observation with reports from others to provide convincing pictures of success. The first report is unsystematic in coverage but seizes on dramatic detail. The second covers a range of settings and people meticulously. Lazarus, Gavillo and Moore (1983), Lindblad-Goldberg (1986), Holmbeck and Lavigne (1992) and Pigott and Gonzales (1987) drew only upon reports from others and covered key aspects of their clients' social functioning in school. These examples show that follow-up enquiries can be conducted economically and quickly, e.g. on the telephone. Where such enquiries are repeated over time, readers can have greater confidence in the validity of the reports (e.g. Imich, 1987).

Sluckin, Foreman and Herbert (1991) followed up a series of children through teacher questionnaires that were distributed between 2 and 10 years after referral. In some recent studies greater use has been made of structured rating instruments to make more systematic data available. For example, 6 months after an intervention for a 6-year-old girl, Powell and Dalley (1995) had the parents and class teacher complete a behaviour rating scale (Burk) and a problem behaviour inventory (Walker) in order to demonstrate that none of the scores reached 'problematic' levels.

In earlier reports key information was often omitted. For example, the report from Lazarus and his colleagues raises more questions than it answers: When did the follow-up enquiries take place? Who were the informants? Why was Karen placed in a clinical day treatment program the following year, and did this relate in any way to her previous difficulties? The information from Lindblad-Goldberg is clear about the child as far as it goes, but it does not cover the other key element of her therapeutic focus – the functioning of the family as a family, the relationships between Jerry and his mother and between Jerry and his stepfather (see the discussion of family therapy in Chapter 5). It may not always be necessary or appropriate for follow-up reports to be based on direct observation of a repeat of the original treatment situation, but they should always provide clear information on the timing of the enquiry and the basis that the informant had for the judgments that are reported. In addition, as far as possible they should address the full range of issues that were highlighted in the original assessment and in the treatment programme, e.g. behaviour difficulties associated with mutism, communication and relationships within the family. If a grid based on the Appendix to this book has been used in the original assessment, it may be helpful to use the same grid for follow-up purposes.

There is very little information available on outcome in adulthood. Periodically over the years Crumley (1990) followed up by phone a child who had been treated at the age of 8, and interviewed him with his parents at the age of 29. The young man was then able to talk revealingly about his feelings and motives in remaining selectively silent as a child. In a more ambitious study Wergeland (1979) reported in detail on a cohort of young adults who had been selectively mute in childhood. His data are impressive in that he succeeded in tracing all 11 people who had been referred for the condition to the children's psychiatric clinic of the University of Oslo between 1955 and 1970. The weakness of his material is that the methods of intervention that had been employed some years earlier are not fully described. They appear, in any case, not to have been satisfactory: an untreated group (who had not received inpatient care because their parents had refused it or for some other reason) had fared better than the group who had been admitted to the clinic. It is to be hoped that, as more investigators begin to conduct long-term follow-up studies now, they may obtain more positive results than were found for the inpatient care that was offered to a previous generation of selectively mute children.

Early indications from the survey evidence that is now becoming available are that those who have been selectively mute in childhood are at risk for continuing problems of communication in adulthood. For example, half of the adults in the survey by Ford et al. (1998) still showed a pattern of selective mutism, a third still found it an effort to speak in certain places, almost half still found it an effort to speak to certain people, and almost half felt uncomfortable in social gatherings, large or small.

As we noted in Chapters 2 and 3, some investigators have begun to treat selective mutism as a developmental subtype of social phobia with earlier onset. In support of that position they have highlighted anecdotal evidence that children who are selectively mute at some stage may continue to show symptoms of social anxiety in later life. Bergman, Piacentini and McCracken (2002) went further and cast doubt on the accepted practice of making a firm distinction between transient and persistent selective mutism. When we discussed the definition of selective mutism at the beginning of this book, we emphasized that a transient refusal of speech in a new situation is usually treated as a brief episode of no developmental significance. These authors drew attention to the fact that there is little empirical evidence to support this assumption and argued that 'if selective mutism represents an early manifestation of social anxiety or an index of behavioural inhibition, then a relatively brief period of mutism could be the initial presentation of a more enduring problem rather than an isolated short-term disorder' (p. 940). If follow-up studies in the future cover a fuller range of developmental sequelae of selective mutism, we will have a stronger empirical basis on which to evaluate such claims.

Reflecting on the extensive work that we have reviewed in this book, we must end with a sobering observation. An important element of follow-up research in the future will be the investigation of the perspectives on selective mutism of previous 'silence users'. The voices of people who have been selectively mute are still largely missing from follow-up reports – and, in fact, from the literature on the subject as a whole.

Appendix 1
Collecting information for assessment

These appendices relate closely to the approach to assessment proposed in Chapter 7. Appendix 1 provides two aids to help plan and conduct interviews. The first is for use when interviewing members of the child's family and the second for use in nursery or school. These lists should be used selectively, according to the needs of an individual case. It is not intended that all the topics that are listed should be covered in any single interview or in any single case. The lists may act as a convenient point of reference in making a decision on what lines of enquiry may be useful in a particular situation. (For a different approach to this task, see Johnson and Wintgens 2001, Chapter 4.)

Information from the family

1. Defining the family/household in relation to selective mutism

You may find it helpful to draw a genogram or family tree with this information shown on it.

- Identify who lives with the child.
- Identify any members of the extended family who see the child often or otherwise play a significant role in her life.
- Identify anyone in these groups who is now selectively mute or very quiet or shy with other people or who has been like that in the past.
- Check how long the family has lived in the area and explore social and communal networks (e.g. parents' participation in social activities outside the home and contact with members of their extended family, with neighbours, and with parents of other children).

2. Early history, habits and temperament

Developmental milestones

- Any developmental milestones where she seemed particularly advanced or late compared to other children in the family (e.g. in crawling, dressing independently, drinking from a cup, etc.)?

Sleeping

- Sleeping situation (room on own/shared with siblings/parents), readiness to go to bed, night fears, sleeping style (sound/interrupted/troubled).

Reaction to change or to something unfamiliar

- In response to something unfamiliar does she most commonly approach it, withdraw from it or stand still and freeze?
- How do you prepare her for new experiences?
- Have you moved house recently/often/once/never?

Separation and loss

- Loss of family members or family friends, through moving home or bereavement, to whom the child was close.
- Separations from mother, father or family in the past, including any illnesses or accidents for which she had to stay in hospital. (For how long? How often? How old was she when this happened? Were her parents able to stay with her?)
- Has the child's mother or father been in hospital? If so, was this a planned admission or an unexpected emergency? How did she react?

- Could she be left with a relative or friend on occasions when the parents had to go somewhere without her? If so, with whom did she like to be left?

Identify any problems in the past or now with:

- Eating habits? Fussy eater? Behaviour at meal times?
- Toilet training? Enuresis? Soiling?
- Fears? Any special incidents which have frightened her (or parents) in the past?
- Any intense fears now (e.g. of the dark/big dogs/thunderstorms)?
- Going to see the doctor?

Upsets and tantrums

- What used to make her get very angry or upset in the past?
- What upsets her now?
- How does she show she is upset?
- What seems to make her anxious?

3. Speech and language

The grid on p. 222 will enable you to summarize the child's speech and language to others. Extensive discussion and some probing may be needed to ensure that a full record is made of the child's verbal and non-verbal communication across settings and across people – at home, in the extended family, and in the neighbourhood. There are some points that it will not be possible to record in the format of the grid. For example:

- What languages other than English are spoken at home or in the extended family? By whom? What attitude does the child have to the use of these languages?
- Was there anything unusual about:

  - her babbling as a baby?
  - the age when she said her first words?
  - the early development of her speech?

- When she started to talk did she mispronounce words at all or have an unusual accent or speak unclearly? Was she ever teased by anyone about her speech?
- Has she seen a speech and language therapist or received any other extra help with speech and language?
- Would she speak to people who came to the house but were not family, e.g. a health visitor?
- Does she communicate with anyone entirely non-verbally – through eye contact, use of gesture, touch, sign language? In what settings? To whom? For what purpose? What are her preferred methods/signs?

- Has she always been shy/selectively mute? Was there a time when she talked normally to a wider range of people than she does now? Can the parents identify any particular event that might have precipitated the change? During this enquiry it may be helpful to emphasize that there is often no specific precipitating event, the onset is often slow and insidious, and it is often difficult for parents thinking back to identify exactly when they noticed that the child was no longer talking to people outside a small circle.

4. Interaction and relationships at home and outside

- Is she especially close to/dependent on/shy of/hostile to/dismissive of mother or father or any particular sibling?
- Is she especially close to/trusting of any adult or child in the extended family or among the parents' friends?
- At home does she like to play in the house/garden/street/playground/in other children's houses? Who does she most like to play with?
- Does she have any friends from nursery/school whom she sees outside school?
- Did she go to playgroup or nursery? Did she settle quickly/slowly? Did she like going?

5. Attitudes and involvement of parents and family

- Attitudes of the mother, father, siblings, other members of the household to her selective mutism?
- Who talks/plays with her at home?
- Availability of key family members for any treatment initiative outside the home, e.g. at school? Willingness to be involved in an initial meeting with teachers (and perhaps in further work)?

6. Progress at school

- Compare her progress at nursery/playgroup and school with that of other children in the family or other children whom the parents know.
- Problems/progress with reading or with learning in general?
- Has her attendance been regular? Does she ever resist going to school?

7. Special interests and 'rewards'

- What activities and games does she most enjoy (e.g. drawing, reading, playing on her bike, playing with toys/dolls/pets, playing outside)?
- Check what her favourite foods and snacks are now (in case this is relevant to suggesting the reinforcement to be used in a treatment plan).

- Are there any strong individual preferences or interests that she shows besides these?

Information from the school

The chief informant will be the child's present class teacher, but some of the information will be available only from school records, and some will be available from others who have taught the child in the past. In the case of selective mutism the observations of nursery assistants and support staff who see the child outside the classroom may be of particular value to supplement the class teacher's perspective.

1. Basic information

- Include ethnicity and languages spoken in the household as recorded at school. Also comment on the speech, use of language, and social relationships in school of any siblings who have attended the same school.

2. Previous school/related experience

- Nursery or other preschool experience? Records/reports about her at that time?
- Has she attended any previous schools? Records/reports?
- School health records? Reports from speech therapist, health visitor or any other professionals available?

3. History in present school

- Date of entry to school
- Discussion with parents before child started?
- Child's behaviour on pre-entry visit to school? During first few days at school?
- Record of speech, language, social interaction, and educational progress in previous classes.
- When was mutism first noted?
- Any earlier interventions to overcome mutism (including informal and short-lived attempts within school) – When? by whom? What kind of intervention? With what result?
- What have the parents' views been when discussing the child with the headteacher or the class teacher?

4. Class teacher's observations on child's communication and interaction

- If she speaks to anyone at school, does she speak normally, in a whisper, briefly or reluctantly?
- List the people to whom she speaks and in what setting (e.g. classroom, playground, cloakroom, hall). Do any special conditions apply (e.g. speaks only when she cannot be overheard or seen by an adult)?
- In the classroom does she seem to listen to the teacher/assistant? Does she make eye contact?
- If she wants something (e.g. a pencil) or wants to do something (e.g. go to the toilet), how does she communicate that – through gesture, by touching the teacher, taking her hand, pointing, bringing her book to her or in some other way?
- If she is engaged in an activity or playing with another child, when the teacher approaches, does she continue, stop, move away?
- When she speaks, is there any indication of a speech difficulty?
- Does she communicate with anyone entirely non-verbally – through eye contact, use of gesture, touch, sign language? In what settings? To whom? For what purpose? What are her preferred methods/signs?
- Has there been any change over time in the pattern of her mutism? E.g. does she speak to more or fewer children/adults than 6/12 months ago/than when she first entered school?

5. Social interaction and educational progress

- Do any of these adjectives describe her behaviour in the classroom: happy, shy, busy, fearful, at ease, passive, anxious, quiet, bold, obstinate, bossy, lively, self-conscious, noisy, unpredictable, watchful? Are there other words that describe her behaviour better?
- Do any of those adjectives describe her behaviour outside the classroom (e.g. in the playground, hall, at lunch time)? In addition, could she be described by any of the following in any of those settings: active, shy, dominating, bullied, aggressive, timid, lively, wild, solitary, slow, disobedient? Add any other words which apply.
- Does she play with other children and/or watch them? If so, where does this take place? Do (some) other children like her, protect her, speak for her, avoid her?
- In the playground does she play with and at lunch time does she sit with – the same children regularly, with different children on different occasions, by herself? Only with girls, only with boys, or with both girls and boys?
- How well is she learning? What areas is she doing best/worst in? Are there special arrangements for getting round her refusal to speak (e.g. reading into a tape-recorder, pointing to correct word to demonstrate reading comprehension)?

6. Special interests and 'rewards'

- What activities and games in school does she like best?
- Which adult(s) in school does she seem to prefer? How does she show this (e.g. by smiling, standing close by in the playground, showing personal possessions, seeking out if she is hurt)?
- Are there any strong individual preferences or interests that she shows besides these?

Appendix 2
A summary record of a child's speech across settings and people

The grid that follows may be used as a summary record sheet for recording where a child speaks and to whom. The use of the simplest form of this grid may be studied in Table 7.3 where it is applied to Maria (aged 4). A more elaborate annotation may be employed to give information not only on where and to whom the child speaks, but also on such issues as frequency, spontaneity and loudness. The greater complexity of this notation may make it appear formidable, but that also increases the amount of information it conveys, which makes it more useful as a vehicle for summarizing progress. As noted in Chapter 7, it may be helpful to give the parents a copy of an (easily intelligible) version of the summary record that is made.

Summary of a child's habits of speech across settings

Child's name:

Places	Own home	Relative's home[a]	Community setting 1[a]	Community setting 2[a]	School setting 1[a]	School setting 2[a]
Date:						
People Mother						
Father						
Sibling 1[b]						
Sibling 2[b]						
Relative 1[b]						
Relative 2[b]						
Teacher[b]						

Completing the summary grid

a Write in the particular settings which are felt to be significant. For example, for Maria (described in Chapter 7) these were her aunt's house, church, park, shops. For Tom (described in Chapter 6) the key school settings seem to have included two different kindergarten classes, the playground and the school bus.

b Write in the name/relationship of the person concerned, e.g.

Mrs Jones, class teacher
Uncle Frank
John, friend/neighbour

Note that some cells have been left blank to allow for different options to be inserted according to the circumstances of the child. In one case some years ago these cells were used for a child's foster mother and foster father, together with one of the other children fostered with the family. In the case of Sara (described in Chapter 5) a cell might have been allocated to her pet parakeet.

Notation

*	Speaks normally
R	Replies to questions and conversational initiatives from others. Does not speak spontaneously on own initiative.
NV	Communicates with this person in this setting only non-verbally, e.g. through pointing, nodding or shaking head or other gestures.
F+	Speaks more frequently than the average child to this person in this setting. (F++ would be more extreme.)
F=	Speaks about as frequently as the average child to this person in this setting.
F–	Speaks less frequently than the average child to this person in this setting. (F– – would be more extreme.)
V	Volume/loudness of voice in everyday speech. V+, V= and V– may be used in the same way as F+, F= and F–.
W	Whispering.
N/A	Not applicable (e.g. for a relative who never visits the child's school a cell relating to the school setting might be completed N/A.)

For an approach to this task that is visually more interesting but does not record quite so much information, see the discussion of a Talking Map by Johnson and Wintgens (2001, pp. 71–73). An advantage of that approach is that children themselves can be given a copy of the 'map' and record their own habits of speech.

Appendix 3
A simple guide to audio feedback treatment

This guide is based on the method used by Nathan Blum, Peter Dowrick and their colleagues in Philadelphia (Blum et al., 1998).

1. In consultation with the child's parents, develop a list of 10–15 open-ended questions about topics that interest the child and are likely to result in more than one-word answers. For example, they used the question, 'what do you like to do with mommy?'
2. Explain to the child the purpose of the audio recordings. They said that it was 'so you can hear what it will be like when you can talk to [here they gave the name of the target person to whom the child did not talk at that time]'.
3. Select 10–15 of the questions and make an audiotape at home of the child answering these questions when they are asked by a parent or someone they talk to easily at home.
4. Make a separate audiotape of the person to whom the child is not talking (the target person) asking the same 10–15 questions.
5. Edit these two audiotapes together to create an intervention audiotape that shows the child giving answers in the context of questions asked by the target person.
6. Establish a baseline by having the target person ask the child the same questions in the setting where they normally meet such as the classroom. Probably there will be no oral response.
7. The parents should now have the child listen to the new audiotape at least twice a day for a week.
8. At the end of the week the target person should again ask the child the questions on the audiotape in the setting where they normally meet. The responses may initially be very quiet, or the child may only answer some of the questions. If so, repeat step 7 for a further period and try again.

Appendix 4
Resources and publications in English

Books

Elective Mutism: A Handbook for Educators, Counsellors and Health Care Practitioners, by Norman H. Hadley

This book, which was written in Canada in 1994, sets out to be eclectic and does indeed cover a wide range of topics around selective mutism. A notable feature of the text is its detailed discussion of the psychological characteristics of silence. Hadley's preferred term for selectively mute people is 'silence users'.

The Selective Mutism Resource Manual by Maggie Johnson and Alison Wintgens

This ring-bound manual, which was published in Britain in 2001, brings together perspectives from two speech and language therapists working in different services: child and adolescent mental health and community health. Their approach is based on behavioural principles and on the notion of a hierarchy of confident speaking. The manual includes detailed and lengthy interview forms and assessment tools.

Refusal to Speak: Treatment of Selective Mutism in Children, edited by Sheila A. Sparaso and Charles E. Schaefer (1999)

This book presents a wide-ranging and eclectic collection of papers from the past and will be useful to researchers and postgraduate students who wish to sample the literature on the treatment of selective mutism without obtaining numbers of journal articles through inter-library loan.

Selective Mutism: Implications for Research and Practice by Thomas S. Kratochwill and colleagues

A revised textbook on selective mutism is in preparation by Thomas Kratochwill of the University of Wisconsin-Madison and his colleagues. It will build on the research they have reported in recent years, much of which has been outlined in this book. The publishers will be Guilford Press of New York.

Support groups

UK

Selective Mutism Information and Research Association (SMIRA)
Contact address: 13 Humberstone Drive, Leicester LE5 0RE
Telephone: 0116 212 7411
E-mail: smiraleicester@hotmail.com

Smira was established in 1992 as a charitable organization that would offer support and advice to parents, teachers, speech therapists, psychologists and other interested professionals. The association holds meetings in Leicester, has regional parent representatives and publishes a newsletter.

USA

Selective Mutism Foundation
Website: www.selectivemutismfoundation.org

This non-profit organization, which was founded in 1991 by two parents of children experiencing selective mutism, aims to provide education, support and research in this area. There have been some recent changes in contact arrangements for the organization, so readers are recommended to check for contact details on the website which offers a wide range of information and links

Selected websites

Selective Mutism Foundation (USA):
http://www.selectivemutismfoundation.org

Selective Mutism Group – Childhood Anxiety Network (USA)
(includes an open discussion forum):
www.childhoodanxietynetwork.org

Essex County Council guidelines for schools:
www.essexcc.gov.uk/educat/parents/specialedneeds/electivemutism.asp

A rare individual hospital/professional site that has extensive support material:
www.quietroom.homestead.com

References

Adams MS (1970) A case of elective mutism. Journal of the National Medical Association 62(3): 213–216.

Adams H, Glasner P (1954) Emotional involvements in some forms of mutism. Journal of Speech and Hearing Disorders 19: 59–69.

Adkins PG (1975) Tina talks. Academic Therapy XI(1): 91–96.

Afnan S, Carr A (1989) Interdisciplinary treatment of a case of elective mutism. British Journal of Occupational Therapy 52(2): 61–66.

Aigen K (1990) Echoes of silence. Music Therapy 9(1): 44–61.

Akhtar S, Buckman J (1977) The differential diagnosis of mutism: a review and a report of three unusual cases. Diseases of the Nervous System 38: 558–562.

Albert EM (1964) Rhetoric, logic and poetics in Burundi: culture patterning of speech behaviour. American Anthropologist 66(6): 35–54.

Albert-Stewart PL (1986) Positive reinforcement in short–term treatment of an electively mute child: a case study. Psychological Reports 58: 571–576.

Ambrosino V, Alessi M (1979) Elective mutism: fixation and the double bind. American Journal of Psychoanalysis 39(3): 251–256.

Andersson CB, Thomsen PH (1998) Electively mute children: an analysis of 37 Danish cases. Nordic Journal of Psychiatry 52(3): 231–238.

Anstendig K (1998) Selective mutism: a review of the treatment literature by modality from 1980–1996. Psychotherapy 35(3): 381–391.

Anstendig KD (1999) Is selective mutism an anxiety disorder? Rethinking its DSM-IV classification. Journal of Anxiety Disorders 13(4): 417–434.

APA (1987) Diagnostic and Statistical Manual of Mental Disorders (3rd edition, Revised) (DSM-III-R). Washington DC: American Psychiatric Association.

APA (1994) Diagnostic and Statistical Manual of Mental Disorders (4th edition) (DSM-IV). Washington, DC: American Psychiatric Association.

Arajarvi T (1965) Elective mutism in children. Annals of Clinical Research of the Finnish Medical Society 11: 46–52.

Atlas JA (1993) Symbol use in a case of elective mutism. Perceptual and Motor Skills 76: 1079–1082.

Atoynatan TH (1986) Elective mutism: involvement of the mother in the treatment of the child. Child Psychiatry and Human Development 17(1): 15–27.

Austad LS, Sininger R, Stricken A (1980) Successful treatment of a case of elective mutism. The Behavior Therapist 3: 18–19.

Ayllon T, Kelly K (1974) Reinstating verbal behavior in a functionally mute retardate. Professional Psychology 385–393.

Baldwin S (1985) No silence please. Times Educational Supplement, 8 November, p. 25.

Baldwin S, Cline T (1991) Helping children who are selectively mute. Educational and Child Psychology 8(3): 72–83.

Bandura A (1969) Principles of Behavior Modification. New York: Holt, Rinehart and Winston.

Bandura A (1977) Self-efficacy: toward a unifying theory of behavioral change. Psychological Review 84: 191–215.

Barlow K, Strother J, Landreth G (1986) Sibling group play therapy: an effective alternative with an elective mute child. The School Counsellor 34(1): 44–50.

Bassey M (1999) Case Study Research in Educational Settings. Buckingham: Open University Press.

Basso K (1970) To give up on words: silence in the Western Apache culture. In: Giglioli P (ed.), Language and Social Context, Harmondsworth: Penguin, pp. 67–86.

Bauermeister JJ, Jemail JA (1975) Modification of 'elective mutism' in the classroom setting – a case study. Behavior Therapy 6(2): 246–250.

Bayley S, Hirst S (1991) A child who did not speak at school: the constructive use of a support worker for behaviour. Maladjustment and Therapeutic Education 9(2): 104–110.

Beck JR, Hubbard MG (1987) Elective mutism in a missionary family. Journal of Psychology and Theology 15(4): 291–299.

Bednar R (1974) A behavioral approach to treating an elective mute in the school. Journal of School Psychology 12: 326–337.

Beidel DC, Randall J (1994) Social phobia. In: Ollendick TH, King NJ, Yule W (eds.), International Handbook of Phobic and Anxiety Disorders in Children and Adolescence. New York: Plenum Press, pp. 111–129.

Beidel DC, Turner SM, Morris TL (1999) Psychopathology of childhood social phobia. Journal of American Academy of Child and Adolescent Psychiatry 38(6): 643–650.

Bergman RL, Piacentini J, McCracken JT (2002) Prevalence and description of selective mutism in a school-based sample. Journal of the American Academy of Child and Adolescent Psychiatry 41(8): 938–946.

Bhide AV, Srinath S (1985) Elective mutism: letter. British Journal of Psychiatry 147: 731.

Black B, Uhde TW (1992) Elective mutism as a variant of social phobia. Journal of American Academy of Child Psychiatry 31(6): 1090–1094.

Black B, Uhde TW (1994) Treatment of elective mutism with fluoxetine: a double-blind, placebo-controlled study. Journal of American Academy of Child Psychiatry 33(7): 1000–1006.

Black B, Uhde TW (1995) Psychiatric characteristics of children with selective mutism: a pilot study. Journal of the American Academy of Child and Adolescent Psychiatry 34(7): 847–856.

Blagg N (1987) School Phobia and its Treatment. London: Routledge.

Blake P, Moss T (1967) The development of socialisation skills in an electively mute child. Behavior Research and Therapy 5: 349–356.

Blanchard EB (1970) The relative contributions of modelling, informational influences and physical contact in the extinction of phobic behavior. Journal of Abnormal Psychology 76: 55–61.

Blatchford P, Sharp S. (eds.) (1994) Breaktime and the School. London: Routledge.

Blotcky MJ, Looney JG (1980) A psychotherapeutic approach to silent children. American Journal of Psychotherapy 24(4): 487–495.

Blum NJ, Kell RS, Starr HL, Lloyds Lender W, Bradley-Klug KL, Osborne ML, Dowrick PW (1998) Case study: audio feedforward treatment of selective mutism. Journal of the American Academy of Child and Adolescent Psychiatry 37(1): 40–43.

Boon F (1994) The selective mutism controversy continued. Journal of the American Academy of Child and Adolescent Psychiatry 33(2): 283.

Bozigar JA, Hansen RA (1984) Group treatment for elective mute children. Social Work 29(5): 478–480.

Bradley S, Sloman L (1975) Elective mutism in immigrant families. Journal of the American Academy of Child Psychiatry 14: 510–514.

Brison DW (1966) A non-talking child in kindergarten: an application of behaviour therapy. Journal of School Psychology 4(4): 65–69.

Brown B, Doll B (1988) Case illustration of classroom intervention with an elective mute child. Special Services in the Schools 5(1–2): 107–125.

Brown B, Lloyd H (1975) A controlled study of children not speaking at school. Journal of the Association of Workers for Maladjusted Children 3: 49–63.

Brown B, Fuller J, Gericke C (1975) Elective mutism: a review and a report of an unsuccessfully treated case. Journal of the Association of Workers for Maladjusted Children 3: 27–37.

Browne E, Wilson V, Laybourne P (1963) Diagnosis and treatment of elective mutism in children. Journal of the American Academy of Child Psychiatry 2: 605–617.

Buck M (1987) An investigation into elective mutism. BEd thesis, Brighton Polytechnic.

Buck M (1988) The silent children. Special Children 22: 12–15.

Busk PL, Serlin RC (1992) Meta-analysis for single-case research. In: Kratochwill TR, Levin JR (eds), Single-Case Research Design and Analysis. Hillsdale, NJ: Lawrence Erlbaum Associates, pp. 187–212.

Calhoun J, Koenig K (1973) Classroom modification of elective mutism. Behavior Therapy 4: 700–702.

Calhoun KS, Turner SM (1981) Historical perspectives and current issues in behavior therapy. In: Turner SM, Calhoun KS, Adams HE (eds), Handbook of Clinical Behavior Therapy. Chichester: Wiley.

Campbell M, Cueva JE (1995) Psychopharmacology in child and adolescent psychiatry: a review of the past seven years. Part II. Journal of the American Academy of Child and Adolescent Psychiatry 34(10): 1262–1272.

Carlson JS, Kratochwill TR, Johnston H (1994) Prevalence and treatment of selective mutism in clinical practice: A survey of child and adolescent psychiatrists. Journal of Child and Adolescent Psychopharmacology 4(4): 281–291.

Carmody L (1999) The power of silence: selective mutism in Ireland – a speech and language therapy perspective. Unpublished dissertation.

Carradice P (1988) Voices in the dorm. Times Educational Supplement, 12 February.

Caspi A, Moffatt TE, Newman DL and Silva PA (1996) Behavioural observation at age 3 years predicts adult psychiatric disorders. Archives of General Psychiatry 53: 1033–1039.

Champernown HI (1963) Art therapy in the Withmead Centre. American Bulletin of Art Therapy Spring issue.

Chapel JL (1970) Behavior modification techniques with children and adolescents. Canadian Psychiatric Association Journal 15: 315–318.

Chau KI (1989) Sociocultural dissonance among ethnic minority populations. Social Casework: The Journal of Contemporary Social Work 224–230.

Chazan M, Laing AF, Davies D, Phillips R (1998) Helping Socially Withdrawn and Isolated Children and Adolescents. London: Cassell.

Chethik M (1975) Amy: the treatment of an elective mute. Journal of the American Academy of Child Psychiatry 12: 482–498.

Ciottone RA, Madonna JM (1984) The treatment of elective mutism: the economics of an integrated approach. Techniques: A Journal for Remedial Education and Counselling, 1 July, 23–30.

Clayton WT (1981) The use of positive reinforcement and stimulus fading in the treatment of elective mutes. Behavioral Psychotherapy 9(2): 25–33.

Cleator HM (1998) Speech and language characteristics of selectively mute children: a speech pathology perspective. Unpublished master's thesis, University of Sydney, Australia.

Cleave S, Jowett S, Bate M (1982) . . . And So To School: A study of continuity from preschool to infant school. Windsor: NFER-Nelson.

Cline T, Kysel F (1987/88) Children who refuse to speak: ethnic background of children with special educational needs described as elective mute. Children and Society 4: 327–334.

Colligan RW, Colligan RC, Dillard MK (1977) Contingency management in the classroom treatment of long–term elective mutism: a case report. Journal of School Psychology 15: 9–17.

Collins J (1996) The Quiet Child. London: Cassell.

Conrad RD, Delk JL, Williams C (1974) Use of stimulus fading procedures in the treatment of situation specific mutism: a case study. Journal of Behaviour Therapy and Experimental Psychiatry 5: 99–109.

Cook JAL (1997) Play therapy for selective mutism. In: Kaduson HG, Cangelosi D, Schaefer CE (eds), The Playing Cure: Individualised Play Therapy for Specific Childhood Problems. Northvale, NJ: Jason Aronson Inc., pp. 83–115.

Cook C, Adams HE (1966) Modification of verbal behavior in speech deficient children. Behavior Research and Therapy 4: 265–271.

Crema JE, Kerr JM (1978) Elective mutism: a child care case study. Child Care Quarterly 7(3): 215–226.

Croghan LM, Craven R (1982) Elective mutism: learning from the analysis of a successful case history. Journal of Pediatric Psychology 7: 85–93.

Crozier WR (2002) Shyness. The Psychologist 15(9): 460–463.

Crumley FE (1990) The masquerade of mutism. Journal of the American Academy of Child and Adolescent Psychiatry 29(2): 318–319.

Crumley FE (1993) Is elective mutism a social phobia? Journal of the American Academy of Child and Adolescent Psychiatry 32(5): 1081.

Cunningham CE, Cataldo MF, Mallion C, Keyes JB (1983) Evaluation of behavioral approaches to the management of elective mutism. Child and Family Behavior Therapy 5(4): 25–49.

Deci EL, Ryan RM (1985) Intrinsic Motivation and Self-Determination in Human Behavior. New York: Plenum Press.

DfES (2000). Standing Order for English Curriculum. See website: http://www.nc.uk.net/nc/contents/En-1-1-POS.html

Dmitriev V, Hawkins J (1973) Suzie never used to say a word. Teaching Exceptional Children 6: 68–76.

Donnelly CL (1998) Anxiety disorders in childhood and adolescence. In: Klykylo WM, Kay J, Rube D (ed), Clinical Child Psychiatry. Philadelphia: WB Saunders, pp. 205–229.

Dow SP, Sonies BC, Scheib D, Moss SE, Leonard HL (1995) Practical guidelines for the assessment and treatment of selective mutism. Journal of the American Academy of Child and Adolescent Psychiatry 34(7): 836–846.

Dowrick PW (1983) Self-modelling. In: Dowrick PW, Biggs SJ (eds), Using Video: Psychological and Social Applications. Chichester: Wiley, pp. 105–124.

Dowrick PW, Hood M (1978) Transfer of talking behaviours across settings using faked films. In: Glynn EL, McNaughton SS (eds), New Zealand Conference for Research in Applied Behavioural Analysis. Auckland, New Zealand: Auckland University Press.

Dummit ES, Klein RG, Tancer NK, Asche B, Martin J (1996) Fluoxetine treatment of children with selective mutism: an open trial. Journal of American Academy of Child and Adolescent Psychiatry 35(5): 615–621.

Dummit ES, Klein RG, Tancer NK, Asche B, Martin J, Fairbanks JA (1997) Systematic assessment of 50 children with selective mutism. Journal of American Academy of Child and Adolescent Psychiatry 36(5): 653–660.

Edmondson C (1986) Elective mutism in children: an examination of its characteristics and remediation. DipSE dissertation, Oxford Polytechnic.

Eldar S, Bleich A, Apter A, Tyano S (1985) Elective mutism antecedent of schizophrenia. Journal of Adolescence 8(3): 289–292.

Elson A, Pearson C, Jones CD, Schumacher E (1965) Follow-up study of childhood elective mutism. Archives of General Psychiatry 13: 182–187.

Ford M, Sladeczek I, Carlson J, Kratochwill TR (1998) Selective mutism: phenomenological characteristics. School Psychology Quarterly 13(3): 192–227.

Friedman R, Karagan N (1973) Characteristics and management of elective mutism in children. Psychology in the Schools 10: 249–252.

Fundudis T, Kolvin I, Garside RF (1979) Speech Retarded and Deaf Children: Their Psychological Development. London: Academic Press.

Furst AL (1989) Elective mutism: report of a case successfully treated by a family doctor. Israel Journal of Psychiatry and Related Sciences 26(1): 96–102.

Gardner PM (1966) Symmetric respect and memorate knowledge: the structure and ecology of individualistic culture. Southwestern Journal of Anthropology 22: 389–415.

Gelfand DM (1979) Social withdrawal and negative emotional states. In:. Wolman BB, Egan J, Ross AO (eds), Handbook on Treatment of Mental Disorders in Childhood. Englewood Cliffs, NJ: Prentice-Hall.

Gemelli RJ (1983) Understanding and helping children who do not talk in school. The Pointer 27(3): 18–23.

Giddan J, Ross GJ, Sechler LL, Becker BR (1997) Selective mutism in elementary school: multidisciplinary intervention. Language, Speech and Hearing Services 28(2): 127–133.

Gillberg C (1996) The long-term outcome of childhood empathy disorders. European Child and Adolescent Psychiatry 5: 52–56.

Goll K (1979) Role structure and subculture in families of elective mute children. Family Process 18: 55–68.

Goll K (1980) Role structure and subculture in families of elective mutists. In: Howells JG (ed.), Advances in Family Psychiatry, New York: International Universities Press, vol. 2, pp. 141–162.

Golwyn DH, Sevlie CP (1999) Phenelzine treatment of selective mutism in four prepubertal children. Journal of Child and Adolescent Psychopharmacology 9: 109–113.

Golwyn DH, Weinstock RC (1990) Phenelzine treatment of elective mutism: a case report. Journal of Clinical Psychiatry 51(9): 384–385.

Graham P, Turk J, Verhulst FC (1999) Child Psychiatry: A Developmental Approach. Oxford: Oxford University Press.

Grannell MT, Hinton SB, O'Kelly SHM (1991) Getting Ready for School: Pack for Parents and Children. Ewell, Surrey: Surrey County Council Education Department.

Gray JA (1987) The Psychology of Fear and Stress (2nd edn). Cambridge: Cambridge University Press.

Gray JA (1988) The neuropsychological basis of anxiety. In: Last C, Hersen M (eds), Handbook of Anxiety Disorders. Elmsford, NY: Pergamon Press, pp. 10–37.

Greenson RR (1961) On the silence and sounds of the analytic hour. Journal of the American Psychoanalytic Association 9: 79–84.

Griffith EE, Schnelle JF, McNees MP, Bissinger C, Huff TM (1975) Elective mutism in a first grader: the remediation of a complex behavioral problem. Journal of Abnormal Child Psychology 2: 127–134.

Guna-Dumitrescu L, Pelletier G (1996) Successful multimodal treatment of a child with selective mutism: A case report (letter to the editor). Canadian Journal of Psychiatry 41(6): 417.

Gupta Y (1990) A case study of an elective mute. Links 15(3): 5–8.

Hadley NH (1994) Elective Mutism: A Handbook for Educators, Counsellors and Health Care Practitioners. Dordrecht: Kluwer.

Hagerman RJ, Hills J, Scahfernaker S, Lewis H (1999) Fragile X syndrome and selective mutism. American Journal of Medical Genetics 83: 313–317.

Halpern WI, Hammond J, Cohen R (1971) A therapeutic approach to speech phobia: elective mutism reexamined. Journal of the American Academy of Child Psychiatry 10(1): 94–107.

Haskell S (1964) Elective mutism (with a case report). In: Renfrew C, Murphy K (eds), The Child Who Does Not Talk. London: Spastics Society/Heinemann Medical, pp. 150–154.

Hayden TL (1980) Classification of elective mutism. Journal of the American Academy of Child Psychiatry 19: 118–133.

Hayden TL (1983) Murphy's Boy. London: Gollancz.

Hayward C, Killen JD, Kraemer HC, Taylor CB (1998) Linking self-reported childhood behavioral inhibition to adolescent social phobia. Journal of American Academy of Child and Adolescent Psychiatry 37(12): 1308–1316.

Hechtman L (1993) Aims and methodological problems in multimodal treatment studies. Canadian Journal of Psychiatry 38(6): 458–464.

Heimlich EP (1981) Patient as assistant therapist in paraverbal therapy with children. American Journal of Psychotherapy 35: 262–267.

Hesse PP (1981) Colour, form and silence: a formal analysis of drawings of a child who did not speak. Arts in Psychotherapy 8: 175–184.

Hesselman S (1983) Elective mutism in children 1877–1981: a literary summary. Acta Paedopsychiatrica 49(6): 297–310.

Heuyer MG, Morgenstern MME (1927) Un cas de mutisme chez un enfant myopathique ancien convulsif. Guérion du mutisme par la psychoanalyse. L'Encéphale 22: 478–481.

Hill L, Scull J (1985) Elective mutism associated with selective inactivity. Journal of Communication Disorders 18: 161–167.

Hoffman S, Laub B (1986) Paradoxical intervention using a polarisation model of cotherapy in the treatment of elective mutism: a case study. Contemporary Family Therapy An International Journal 8(2): 136–143.

Holmbeck GN, Lavigne JV (1992) Combining self-modelling and stimulus fading in the treatment of an electively mute child. Psychotherapy 29: 661–667.

Howard M (1963) Art: a therapeutic tool. Journal of the Oklahoma State Medical Association 56: 420–424.

Hultquist AM (1995) Selective mutism: causes and interventions. Journal of Emotional and Behavioral Disorders 3(2): 100–107.

Imich AJ (1987) Programmed intervention for a child who does not speak in school. Links 13(1): 6–13.

Imich A (1998) Selective mutism: the implications of current research for the practice of educational psychologists. Educational Psychology in Practice 14(1): 52–59.

Inniss J (1977) Counselling the culturally disrupted child. Elementary School Guidance and Counselling 11(3): 229–235.

Jacobsen T (1995) Case study: Is selective mutism a manifestation of dissociative identity disorder? Journal of the American Academy of Child and Adolescent Psychiatry 34(7): 863–866.

Jefferies E, Dolan S (1994) Reluctant talkers in the early years: some key issues. In Watson J (ed.), Working with Communication Difficulties. Edinburgh: Moray House Publications, pp. 106–120.

Jelley D (2000) The internet and a 'small miracle': a patient who changed my practice. British Medical Journal 7254: 165–166.

Johnson C (1987) Seen but not heard: the dilemma of the shy child. Momentum 44–46.

Johnson M, Glassberg AH (1992) Breaking Down the Barriers Created by Selectively Mute Children: A Structured Treatment Plan Written for Speech and Language Therapists and Teachers. Canterbury: Canterbury and Thanet Speech and Language Therapy Department.

Johnson M, Wintgens A (2001) The Selective Mutism Resource Manual. Bicester, Oxfordshire: Speechmark.

Jones MC (1924) Elimination of children's fears. Journal of Experimental Psychology 7: 382–390.

Joseph PR (1999) Selective mutism – the child who doesn't speak at school. Pediatrics 104(2): 308–310.

Kagan J, Reznick JS, Snidman N (1987) The physiology and psychology of behavioral inhibition in children. Child Development 58: 1459–1473.

Kanner L (1947) Child Psychiatry. Springfield, IL: Charles C. Thomas.

Kaplan SL, Escoll P (1973) Treatment of two silent adolescent girls. Journal of the American Academy of Child Psychiatry 12: 59–72.

Kass W, Gillman AE, Mattis AS (1967) Treatment of selective mutism in a blind child: school and clinic collaboration. American Journal of Orthopsychiatry 37: 215–216.

Kazdin AE (1978) History of Behavior Modification: Experimental Foundations of Contemporary Research. Baltimore, MD: University Park Press.

Kazdin AE (1992) Research Design in Clinical Psychology. New York: Macmillan.

Kee CHY, Fung DSS, Ang L (2001) An electronic communication device for selective mutism: letter. Journal of the American Academy for Child and Adolescent Psychiatry 40(4): 389.

Kehle TJ, Owen SV, Cressy ET (1990) The use of self–modelling as an intervention in school psychology: a case study. School Psychology Review 19(1): 115–121.

Kehle TJ, Madaus MR, Baratta VS, Bray MA (1998) Augmented self-modeling as a treatment for children with selective mutism. Journal of School Psychology 36(3): 247–260.

Kelly JA (1981) Using puppets for behaviour rehearsal in social skills training with young children. Child Behavior Therapy 3(1): 61–64.

Kendall PC, Ronan K (1990) Assessment of children's anxieties, fears and phobias: cognitive-behavioral models and methods. In: Reynolds CR, Kamphaus RW (eds.), Handbook of Psychological and Educational Assessment of Children. New York: Guilford Press, vol. 2, pp. 223–244.

Kerr M, Lambert WW, Statin H, Klackenberg-Larsson I (1994) Stability of inhibition in a Swedish longitudinal sample. Child Development 65: 138–146.

Klin A, Volkmar FR (1983) Elective mutism and mental retardation. Journal of the American Academy of Child and Adolescent Psychiatry 32(4): 860–864.

Koch M, Goodlund L (1973) Children who refuse to talk: a follow-up study. Bulletin of the Bell Museum of Pathobiology 2: 30–32.

Kolakowski A, Liwska M, Wolanczyk T (1996) Selective mutism in children – a literature review. Psychiatria Polska XXX(2): 233–246.

Kolvin I, Fundudis T (1981) Elective mute children: psychological development and background factors. Journal of Child Psychology and Psychiatry 22(3): 219–232.

Kopp S, Gillberg C (1997) Selective mutism: A population-based study: A research note. Journal of Child Psychology and Psychiatry 38(2): 257–261.

Kratochwill T (1981) Selective Mutism: Implications for Research and Treatment. Hillsdale, NJ: Lawrence Erlbaum Associates.

Kratochwill TR, Brody G, Piersel W (1979) Elective mutism in children. Advances in Clinical Child Psychology 2: 194–241.

Kristensen H (1997) Elective mutism – associated with developmental disorder/delay. Two case studies. European Child and Adolescent Psychiatry 6: 234–239.

Kristensen H (2000) Selective mutism and comorbidity with developmental disorder/delay, anxiety disorder and elimination disorder. Journal of the American Academy of Child and Adolescent Psychiatry 39(2): 249–256.

Kristensen H (2002) Non-specific markers of neurodevelopmental disorder/delay in selective mutism. A case-control study European Child and Adolescent Psychiatry 11(2): 71–78.

Kristensen H, Torgersen S (2001) MCMI-II personality traits and symptom traits in parents of children with selective mutism: a case-control study. Journal of Abnormal Psychology 110(4): 648–652.

Krohn DD, Weckstein SM, Wright HL (1992) A study of the effectiveness of a specific treatment for elective mutism. Journal of the American Academy of Child and Adolescent Psychiatry 31(4): 711–718.

Krolian EB (1988) 'Speech is silvern, but silence is golden' Day hospital treatment of two electively mute children. Clinical Social Work Journal 16(4): 355–377.

Kumpulainen K, Räsänen E, Raaska H, Somppi V (1998) Selective mutism among second-graders in elementary school. European Child and Adolescent Psychiatry 7: 24–29.

Kupietz S, Schwartz IL (1982) Elective mutism: evaluation and behavioural treatment. New York State Journal of Medicine 82(7): 1073–1076.

Labbe EE, Williamson DA (1984) Behavioral treatment of elective mutism: a review of the literature. Clinical Psychology Review 4(3): 273–292.

Lachenmeyer JR, Gibbs MS (1985) The social–psychological functions of reward in the treatment of a case of elective mutism. Journal of Social and Clinical Psychology 3(4): 466–473.

Lafferty J, Constantino JN (1998) Fluvoxamine in selective mutism. Journal of the American Academy of Child and Adolescent Psychiatry 37(1): 12–13.

Landgarten H (1975) Art therapy as primary mode of treatment for an elective mute. American Journal of Art Therapy 14: 121–125.

Larsson DG, Larsson EV (1983) Manipulating peer prescence to program the generalisation of verbal compliance from one-to-one to group instruction. Education and Treatment of Children 6(2): 109–122.

Last CG, Perrin S, Hersen M, Kazdin AE (1992) DSM-III-R anxiety disorders in children: sociodemographic and clinical characteristics. Journal of the American Academy of Child and Adolescent Psychiatry 31, 1070–6.

Lazarus PJ, Gavillo HM, Moore JW (1983) The treatment of elective mutism in children within the school setting: two case studies. School Psychology Review 12(4): 467–472.

Lebrun Y (1990) Mutism. London: Whurr.

Leonard H, Dow S (1995) Selective Mutism. In: March JS (ed.), Anxiety Disorders in Children and Adolescents. New York: Guilford Press, pp. 235–250.

Leonard HL, Topol DA (1993) Elective mutism. Child and Adolescent Psychiatric Clinics of North America 2(4): 695–707.

Lepper MR, Gilovich T (1981) The multiple functions of reward: a social-developmental perspective. In: Brehm SS, Kassin SM, Gibbons FX (eds), Developmental Social Psychology. New York: Oxford University Press.

Lesser-Katz M (1986) Stranger reaction and elective mutism in young children. American Journal of Orthospychiatry 56(3): 458–469.

Lindblad-Goldberg M (1986) Elective mutism in families with young children. In: Combrinck-Graham L (ed.), Treating Young Children in Family Therapy. Rockville Maryland: Aspen, vol. 18, pp. 31–42.

Lipton H (1980) Rapid reinstatement of speech using stimulus fading with a selectively mute child. Journal of Behavior Therapy and Experimental Psychiatry 11: 147–149.

Looff DH (1971) Appalachia's Children: The Challenge of Mental Health. Lexington, KY: University Press of Kentucky.

Louden DM (1987) Elective mutism: a case study of a disorder of childhood. Journal of the National Medical Association 79(10): 1043–1048.

Lovaas OI, Berberich JP, Perloff BF, Schaeffer B (1966) Acquisition of imitative speech by schizophrenic children. Science 51: 705–707.

Lowenstein LF (1979) The result of twenty-one elective mute cases. Acta Paedopsychiatrica 45: 17–23.

Lumb D, Wolff D (1988) Mary doesn't talk. British Journal of Special Education 15(3): 103–106.

Lysne A (1995) Elective mutism: special treatment of a special case. Scandinavian Journal of Educational Research 39(2): 93–97.

Lytton H, Conway D, Sauve R (1977) The impact of twinship on parent–child interaction. Journal of Personality and Social Psychology 35(2): 97–107.

McGregor R, Pullar A, Cundall D (1994) Silent in school – elective mutism and abuse. Archives of Disease in Childhood 70(6): 540–541.

McGrew WC (1972) Aspects of social development in nursery school children with emphasis on introduction to the group. In: Burton Jones N (ed), Ethological Studies of Child Behaviour. Cambridge: Cambridge University Press.

Mack JR, Maslin B (1981) The facilitating effect of claustral experience on the speech of psychogenically mute children. Journal of the American Academy of Child Psychiatry 20: 65–70.

Malmstrom PM, Silva MN (1986) Twin talk: manifestations of twin status in the speech of toddlers. Journal of Child Language 13: 293–304.

Maskey S (2001) Selective mutism, social phobia and moclobemide: a case report. Clinical Child Psychology and Psychiatry 6(3): 363–369.

Masten WG, Stacks JR, Caldwell-Colbert AT, Jackson JS (1996) Behavioral treatment of a selective mute Mexican-American boy. Psychology in the Schools 33: 56–60.

Matson JL (1981) Assessment and treatment of clinical fears in mentally retarded children. Journal of Applied Behavior Analysis 14: 287–294.

Matson JL, Esveldt-Dawson K, O'Donnell D (1979) Overcorrection, modeling, and reinforcement procedures for reinstating speech in a mute boy. Child Behavior Therapy 1(4): 363–371.

Meijer A (1979) Elective mutism in children. Israel Annals of Psychiatry and Related Disciplines 17: 93–100.

Meyers SV (1984) Elective mutism in children: a family systems approach. American Journal of Family Therapy 22(4): 39–45.

Mora G, De Vault S, Schopler E (1962) Dynamics and psychotherapy of identical twins with elective mutism. Journal of Child Psychology and Psychiatry 3: 41–52.

Morin C, Ladouceur R, Cloutier R (1982) Reinforcement procedures in the treatment of reluctant speech. Journal of Behaviour Therapy and Experimental Psychiatry 13: 145–147.

Morris JV (1953) Cases of elective mutism. American Journal of Mental Deficiency 57: 661–668.

Motavalli N (1995) Fluoxetine for (s)elective mutism. Journal of the American Academy of Child and Adolescent Psychiatry 34(6): 701–702.

Munford PR, Reardon D, Liberman RP, Allen L (1976) Behavioral treatment of hysterical coughing and mutism: a case study. Journal of Consulting and Clinical Psychology 44: 1008–1014.

Myquel M, Granon M (1982) Le mutisme électif extrafamiliale chez l'enfant. Neuropsychiatrie de l'Enfance et de l'Adolescence 30(6): 329–339.

Nash R, Thorpe H, Andrews M, Davis K (1979) A management program for elective mutism. Psychology in the Schools 16(2): 246–253.

Nolan JD, Pence C (1970) Operant conditioning principles in the treatment of a selectively mute child. Journal of Counselling and Clinical Psychology 35(2): 265–268.

Norman A, Broman HJ (1970) Volume feedback and generalisation techniques in shaping speech of an electively mute boy: a case study. Perceptual and Motor Skills 31: 463–470.

Oosterlaan J (2001) Behavioural inhibition and the development of childhood anxiety disorders. In: Silverman WK, Treffers P (eds.), Anxiety Disorders in Children and Adolescents: Research Assessment and Intervention. Cambridge: Cambridge University Press, pp. 45–71.

Paniagua FA, Saeed MA (1987) Labelling and functional language in a case of psychological mutism. Journal of Behavior Therapy and Experimental Psychiatry 18(3): 259–267.

Paniagua FA, Saeed MA (1988) A procedural distinction between elective and progressive mutism. Journal of Behavior Therapy and Experimental Psychiatry 19: 207–210.

Parker EB, Olsen TF, Throckmorton MC (1960) Social case work with elementary school children who do not talk in school. Social Work 5: 64–70.

Pecukonis EV, Pecukonis MT (1991) An adapted language training strategy in the treatment of an electively mute child. Journal of Behavior Therapy and Experimental Psychiatry 22(1): 9–21.

Phelps L, Brown RT, Power TJ (2002) Pediatric Psychopharmacology: Combining Medical and Psychosocial Interventions. Washington, DC: American Psychological Association.

Piersel WC, Kratochwill TR (1981) A teacher implemented contingency management package to assess and treat selective mutism. Behavioural Assessment 3: 371–382.

Pigott HE, Gonzales FP (1987) Efficacy of video tape self-modelling in treating an electively mute child. Journal of Clinical Child Psychology 16(2): 106–110.

Pine DS, Grun J (1998) Anxiety disorders. In: Walsh BT (ed.), Child Psychopharmacology. Washington, DC: American Psychiatric Press, pp. 115–148.

Porjes MD (1992) Intervention with the selectively mute child. Psychology in the Schools 29: 367–376.

Powell S, Dalley M (1995) When to intervene in selective mutism: the multimodal treatment of a case of persistent selective mutism. Psychology in the Schools 32: 114–123.

Prins PJM (2001) Affective and cognitive processes. In: Silverman WK, Treffers PDA (eds.), Anxiety Disorders in Children and Adolescents. Cambridge: Cambridge University Press.

Prior M (1992) Childhood temperament. Journal of Child Psychology and Psychiatry 33(1): 249–280.

Pustrom E, Speers RW (1964) Elective mutism in children. Journal of Child Psychiatry 3: 287–297.

Radford P (1977) A study of an elective mute. In: Boston M, Daws D (eds), The Child Psychotherapist and the Problems of Young People. London: Wildwood House, pp. 160–182.

Rapoport JL, Ismond DR (1996) DSM-IV Training Guide for Diagnosis of Childhood Disorders. New York: Brunner/Mazel.

Rasbury WC (1974) Behavioral treatment of selective mutism: a case report. Journal of Behavior Therapy and Experimental Psychiatry 5: 103–104.

Reed GF (1963) Elective mutism in children: a reappraisal. Journal of Child Psychology and Psychiatry 4: 99–107.

Reid JB, Hawkins N, Keutzer C, McNeal SA, Phelps RE, Mees HL (1967) A marathon behaviour modification of a selectively mute child. Journal of Child Psychology and Psychiatry 8: 27–30.

Reznick JS, Hegeman IM, Kaufman ER, Woods SW, Jacobs M (1992) Retrospective and concurrent self-support of behavioural inhibition and their relation to adult mental health. Development and Psychopathology 4: 301–21.

Richards S, Hansen M (1978) A further demonstration of the efficacy of stimulus fading treatment of elective mutism. Journal of Behavior Therapy and Experimental Psychiatry 9: 57–60.

Richburg ML, Cobia DC (1994) Using behavioral techniques to treat elective mutism: a case study. Elementary School Guidance and Counselling 28(3): 214–210.

Rigby MA (1929) A case of lack of speech due to negativism. Psychological Clinics 18: 156–161.

Roberts J (1984) Switching models: family and team choice points and reactions as we moved from the Haley strategic model to the Milan model. Journal of Strategic and Systemic Therapies 3(4): 40–53.

Roe V (1993) An interactive therapy group. Child Language Teaching and Therapy 9(2): 133–140.

Rosenbaum E, Kellman M (1973) Treatment of a selectively mute third grade child. Journal of School Psychology 11: 26–29.

Rosenberg JB, Lindblad MB (1978) Behaviour therapy in a family context: treating elective mutism. Family Process 17: 77–82.

Rossouw T, Lubbe T (1994) Psychotherapy of a young boy with elective mutism. Psycho-analytic Psychotherapy in South Africa, Winter issue, 21–30.

Rupp SN (1999) Haloperidol for Tourette's disorder plus selective mutism. Journal of the American Academy of Child and Adolescent Psychiatry 38(1): 7.

Russell PSS, Raj SE, John JK (1998) Multimodal intervention for selective mutism in mentally retarded children. Journal of the American Academy of Child and Adolescent Psychiatry 37(9): 903–904.

Rutter M (1977) Speech delay. In: Rutter M, Hersov L (eds), Child Psychiatry: Modern Approaches. Oxford: Blackwell.

Ruzicka B, Sackin H (1974) Elective mutism: the impact of the patient's silent detachment upon the therapist. Journal of the American Academy of Child Psychiatry 13: 551–561.

Salfield DJ (1950) Observations on elective mutism in children. Journal of Mental Science 96: 1024–1033.

Sanok RL, Ascione FR (1979) Behavioral interventions for childhood elective mutism: an evaluative review. Child Behavior Therapy 1: 49–68.

Sanok R, Striefel S (1979) Elective mutism: generalisation of verbal responding across people and settings. Behavior Therapy 10(3): 357–371.

Savic S (1980) How Twins Learn to Talk: A Study of the Speech Development of Twins from 1 to 3. Translated by Vladislava Felbabov. London: Academic Press.

Saville-Troike M (1982) The Ethnography of Communication: An Introduction. Oxford: Basil Blackwell.

Schachter M (1981) Mutisme électif ou refus électif de parler, chez l'enfant: panorama critique de la literature mondiale de 1934 à 1979. Feuillots Psychiatriques de Liège 14: 490–501.

Schaefer C (ed.) (1993) The Therapeutic Powers of Play. Northvale, NJ: Jason Aronson.

Schill MT, Kratochwill TR, Gardner WI (1996a) Conducting a functional analysis of behavior. In: Breen MJ, Fiedler CR (eds.) Behavioral Approach to Assessment of Youth With Emotional/Behavioral Disorders: A Handbook for School-Based Practitioners. Austin, TX: Pro.Ed.

Schill MT, Kratochwill TR, Gardner WI (1996b) An assessment protocol for selective mutism: analogue assessment using parents as facilitators. Journal of School Psychology 34(1): 1–21.

Schroeder BA (1992) Human Growth and Development. St. Paul, MN: West Publishing.

Scott E (1977) A desensitisation programme for the treatment of mutism in a seven year old girl: a case report. Journal of Child Psychology and Psychiatry 18: 263–270.

Selfe L (2002) Discussion paper – concerns about the identification and diagnosis of autistic spectrum disorders. Educational Psychology in Practice 18(4): 335–341.

Semenoff B, Park C, Smith E (1976) Behavioral interventions with a six year old elective mute. In: Krumbolz JD, Thoresen CE (ed.), Counseling Methods. New York: Holt, Rinehart and Winston, pp. 89–97.

Shaw WH (1971) Aversive control in the treatment of elective mutism. Journal of the American Academy of Child Psychiatry 10: 572–581.

Sheridan SM, Kratochwill TR, Ramirez SZ (1995) Assessment and treatment of selective mutism: recommendations and a case study. Special Services in the Schools 10(1): 55–77.

Shreeve DF (1991) Elective mutism: origins in stranger anxiety and selective attention. Bulletin of the Menninger Clinic 55(4): 491–504.

Shvartzman P, Hornshtein I, Klein E, Yechezkel A, Ziv M, Herman J. (1990) Elective mutism in family practice. Journal of Family Practice 31(3): 319–320.

Silverman G, Powers DG (1970) Elective mutism in children. Medical College of Virginia Quarterly 6: 182–186.

Simons D, Goode S, Fombonne E (1997) Elective mutism and chromosome 18 abnormality. European Child and Adolescent Psychiatry 6: 112–114.

Sluckin A (1977) Children who do not talk at school. Child: Care Health and Development 3: 69–79.

Sluckin A (2000) Selective mutism. In: Law J, Parkinson A, Tamhne R (eds), Communication Difficulties in Childhood: A Practical Guide. Abingdon: Radcliffe Medical Press, pp. 273–280.

Sluckin A, Jehu D (1969) A behavioural approach in the treatment of elective mutism. British Journal of Psychiatric Social Work 10: 70–73.

Sluckin A, Foreman N, Herbert M (1991) Behavioural treatment programs and selectivity of speaking at follow-up in a sample of 25 selective mutes. Australian Psychologist 26(2): 132–137.

Sluzki CE (1983) The sounds of silence: two cases of elective mutism in bilingual families. Family Therapy Collections 6: 68–77.

Smayling JM (1959) Analysis of six cases of voluntary mutism. Journal of Speech and Hearing Disorders 24: 55–58.

Southworth P (1987) Happy talk. Cambridge Journal of Education 17: 156–158.

Southworth P (1988) Happy talk: how Pam Southworth coped with a child who wouldn't speak. Times Educational Supplement, 29 January.

Spence SH, Donovan C, Brechman-Toussaint M (2000) The treatment of childhood social phobia: the effectiveness of a social skills training-based, cognitive-behavioural intervention, with and without parental involvement. Journal of Child Psychology and Psychiatry 41(6): 713–726.

Stein MT, Rapin I, Yapko D (2001) Selective mutism. Pediatrics 107(4): 926–929.

Steinhausen HC, Adamek R (1997) The family history of children with elective mutism: a research report. European Child and Adolescent Psychiatry 6: 107–111.

Steinhausen H, Juzi C (1996) Elective mutism: an analysis of 100 cases. Journal of the American Academy of Child and Adolescent Psychiatry 35(5): 606–614.

Stephenson C (1993) Use of drama. In: Dwivedi KN (ed.), Group Work with Children and Adolescents: A Handbook. London: Jessica Kingsley, pp. 170–182.

Stone BP, Kratochwill TR, Sladezcek I, Serlin RC (2002) Treatment of selective mutism: a best-evidence synthesis. School Psychology Quarterly 17(2): 168–190.

Strait R (1958) A child who was speechless in school and social life. Journal of Speech and Hearing Disorders 23: 253–254.

Straughan JH (1968) The application of operant conditioning to the treatment of elective mutism. In: Sloane HNJ, Macaulay BD (eds), Operant Procedures in Remedial Speech and Language Training. Boston: Houghton Mifflin, pp. 242–255.

Straughan JH, Potter WK Jr, Hamilton SH Jr (1965) The behavioral treatment of an elective mute. Journal of Child Psychology and Psychiatry 6: 125–130.

Subak ME, West M, Carlin M (1982) Elective mutism: an expression of family psychopathology. International Journal of Family Psychiatry 3: 335–344.

Szabo CP (1996) Selective mutism and social anxiety. Journal of the American Academy of Child and Adolescent Psychiatry 35(5): 555.

Tachibana R, Nakamura K, Shichuri K, Usuda S (1982) Elective mutism in identical twins. Japanese Journal of Child and Adolescent Psychiatry 23(5): 277–286.

Tancer NK (1992) Elective mutism: a review of the literature. In: Lahey BB. Kazdin AE (eds.), Advances in Clinical Psychology. New York: Plenum, vol. 14, pp. 265–288.

Tatem D, DelCampo RL (1995) Selective mutism in children: a structural family therapy approach to treatment. Contemporary Family Therapy 17(2): 177–194.

Taylor S, Dossetor DR, Kilham H, Bernard E (2000) The youngest case of pervasive refusal syndrome? Clinical Child Psychology and Psychiatry 5(1): 23–29.

Thomas A, Chess S, Birch HG (1968) Temperament and Behavior Disorders in Children. New York: New York University Press.

Thorpe K, Greenwood R, Eivers A, Rutter M (2001) Prevalence and development of 'secret language'. International Journal of Language and Communication 36: 43–62.

Tibbles PN, Russell G (1992) The silence of symbiosis: the difficulty in separating a silent adolescent daughter and an uncommunicative mother. British Journal of Psychotherapy 8(3): 266–277.

Tittnich E (1990) Clinical illustration: elective mutism. Journal of Children in Contemporary Society 21(1–2): 151–158.

Tomasello M, Mannle S, Kruger AC (1986) Linguistic environment of 1–2-year-old twins. Developmental Psychology 22(2): 169–176.

Tramer M (1934) Electiver Mutismus bei Kindern. Zeitschrift für Kinderpsychiatrie 1: 30–35.

Turner SM, Beidel DC, Wolff PL (1996) Is behavioural inhibition related to anxiety disorders? Clinical Psychology Review 16: 157–172.

Twernbold MA, Kratochwill TR, Gardner WI (1996) An assessment protocol for selective mutism: Analogue assessment using parents as facilitators. Journal of School Psychology 34: 1–21.

Valner J, Nemiroff M (1995) Silent eulogy: elective mutism in a six-year-old Hispanic girl. Psychoanalytic Study of the Child 50: 327–340.

Van der Kooy D, Webster CD (1975) A rapidly effective behaviour modification programme for an electively mute child. Journal of Behaviour Therapy and Experimental Psychiatry 6(2): 149–152.

Vasey MW, Daleiden EL (1996) Information processing pathways to cognitive interference in childhood. In: Sarason IG, Pierce GR, Sarason BR (eds.), Cognitive Interference: Theories Methods and Findings. Hillsdale, NJ: Lawrence Erlbaum Associates, pp. 117–138.

Velting ON, Albino AM (2001) Current trends in the understanding and treatment of social phobia in youth. Journal of Child Psychology and Psychiatry 42(1): 127–140.

Wallace M (1986) The Silent Twins. London: Penguin.

Waller D (1991) Becoming a Profession: The History of Art Therapy in Britain 1940–1982. London: Tavistock/Routledge.

Wassing H (1973) A case of prolonged elective mutism in an adolescent boy: on the nature of the condition and its residential treatment. Acta Paedopsychiatrica 40: 75–96.

Waterman P, Shatz M (1982) The acquisition of personal pronouns and proper names by an identical twin pair. Journal of Speech and Hearing Research 25: 149–154.

Watson S (1995) Successful treatment of selective mutism: collaborative work in a secondary school setting. Child Language Teaching and Therapy 11(2): 163–175.

Watson TS, Kramer JJ (1992) Multimethod behavioral treatment of long-term selective mutism. Psychology in the Schools 29: 359–366.

Weckstein SM, Krohn DD, Wright HL (1995) Elective mutism. In: Eisen AR, Kearney CA, Schaefer CE (eds.) Clinical Handbook of Anxiety Disorders in Children and Adolescents. Northvale, NJ: Jason Aronson, pp. 169–194.

Weininger O (1987) Electively mute children: a therapeutic approach. Journal of the Melanie Klein Society 5(1): 25–42.

Wergeland H (1979) Elective mutism. Acta Psychiatrica Scandinavia 59: 218–228.

WHO (1992) The ICD-10 Classification of Mental and Behavioural Disorders. Geneva: World Health Organization.

Wickings S, Jenkins J, Carr J, Corbett J (1974) Modification of behavior using a shaping procedure. Apex 2(6).

Wilkins R (1985) A comparison of elective mutism and emotional disorders in children. British Journal of Psychiatry 146: 198–203.

Williamson DA, Sewell WR, Sanders SH, Haney JN, White D (1977a). The behavioral treatment of elective mutism: two case studies. Journal of Behavior Therapy and Experimental Psychiatry 8: 143–149.

Williamson DA, Sewell WR, Sanders SH, Haney JN, White D (1977b). The treatment of reluctant speech using contingency management procedures. Journal of Behavior Therapy and Experimental Psychiatry 8: 155–156.

Winter S (1984) Peer therapy for elective mutism. Behavioural Approaches with Children 8(4): 134–137.

Wintgens A (1999) Tackling speech and language when assessing and treating children with selective mutism. Workshop presentation at the AFASIC Third International Symposium, York.

Wolfendale S (1990) All About Me. Nottingham: NES/Arnold.

Wolpe J (1958) Psychotherapy By Reciprocal Inhibition. Stanford, CA: Stanford University Press.

Woo R (1999) Sounds of silence: the need for presence in absence. Journal of Child Psychotherapy 25(1): 93–114.

Wright HL (1968) A clinical study of children who refuse to talk in school. Journal of the American Academy of Child Psychiatry 7: 603–617.

Wright A (1991) Enhancing motivation in children and adults. In: Wright A, Frederickson N (eds), Developing Self–Discipline. London: Educational Psychology Publishing, University College London.

Wright HH (1994) Selective mutism continued (letter). Journal of the American Academy of Child and Adolescent Psychiatry 33(4): 593.

Wright HH, Miller MD, Cook MA, Littman JR (1985) Early identification and intervention with children who refuse to speak. Journal of the American Academy of Child Psychiatry 24(6): 739–746.

Wright HH, Cuccaro ML, Leonhardt TV, Kendall DF, Anderson JH (1995) Case study: fluoxetine in the multimodal treatment of a preschool child with selective mutism. Journal of the American Academy of Child and Adolescent Psychiatry 34(7): 857–862.

Wulbert M, Nyman BA, Snow D, Owen Y (1973) The efficacy of stimulus fading and contingency management in the treatment of elective mutism. Journal of Applied Behavioral Analysis 6: 435–441.

Yanof J (1996) Language, communication and transference in child analysis: I. Selective mutism: the medium is the message. Is child analysis really analysis? Journal of the American Psychoanalytic Association 44: 79–116.

Yin RK (1994) Case Study Research: Design and Methods (2nd edition). Newbury Park, CA: Sage Publications.

Youngerman J (1979) The syntax of silence: electively mute therapy. International Review of Psychoanalysis 6(3): 283–295.

Zeligs MA (1961) The psychology of silence: its role in the transference, countertransference and the psychoanalytic process. Journal of the American Psychoanalytic Association 9: 7–43.

Author index

Subject index

Printed in the United States
90203LV00001B/23/A